THE STRONG BRAIN

How Neuroscience Explains Addiction, Depression, and the Roots of Psychiatric Disorders

NICOLE V. PIRES

THE STRONG BRAIN

How Neuroscience Explains Addiction, Depression, and the Roots of Psychiatric Disorders

NICOLE V. PIRES

You can find all references at www.thestrongbrain.com

Dedicated to Tia Chica and Vovô Antônio, whom I have loved deeply since the beginning of my existence and to whom this book owes its very being.

Dedicated to Madrinha Fernanda, whose life ended much sooner than we all hoped. This book is the beginning of a legacy built to honor her.

Dedicated to those who are madly in love with life and to those for whom the desire to live has died. I hope that, by the end of this book, the latter find their way to the former.

TABLE OF CONTENTS

Part I: The Foundations of The Sick Brain 7
1. Childhood, Purpose, and the Lost Confidence 8
2. The Modern Mind in Crisis 32
3. What Makes a Brain Sick? 76

Part II. The Major Disorders of Our Time 103
4. Addiction: The Mind's Favorite Poison 105
5. Anxiety: The Overheated Brain 119
6. Depression: The Silent Void of Sadness and Suicide 151

Part III - Forces Driving the Collapse 174
7. Cancel Culture and Negativity 176
8. The Brain Will Heal if You Let It 206

Part IV - Healing the Sick Brain 225
9. Purpose, Connection, and Meaning 227

Part I

The Foundations of The Sick Brain

CHAPTER 1
Childhood, Purpose, and the Lost Confidence

Just as the laws of quantum mechanics do not guarantee a single outcome for every observation, the human mind and body refuse to respond in one fixed way to any given circumstance. Our neurons form countless possible connections, their patterns influenced by subtle shifts in mood, the temperature of the air, the hour of the day, even the faces surrounding us. We have dissected human anatomy with remarkable precision, mapping each organ's function in detail, yet the body's reactions to certain triggers remain mysterious; elusive variables in an equation we cannot yet solve. This inherent unpredictability of our nature is evident from the very start of life, in the capricious emotional worlds of children.

When I was a child, I had two best friends: Marta and Bianca. We lived close to one another, and our after-school afternoons became a long-awaited ritual, rotating from house to house in an endless playdate. We were each an only child, so we filled the role of sisters for one another as soon as the school bell rang. On evenings when it was my turn to host, my mother would bake a batch of *pães de queijo*—warm, cheesy buns whose delicious scent filled our kitchen. We would devour them happily, giggling between bites. At Bianca's house, the highlight of the night was playing with her little dog. And at Marta's home, we often ended the day curled into the living room couch with a movie, or else we would lay down on the floor with a pile of books. Marta especially loved reading; she devoured at least one hefty novel a week even at that young age. (I used to look at that and think, "I could never read all of this!" Now, I am the one writing books, but I guess at that age I was fine just playing with legos.) Looking back, I sense she might have been escaping into those stories, slipping away from a reality that—though I could not name it then—I now understand was marked by chaos in her family life. Each of us found comfort in something: for Marta it was books, for Bianca it was her dog's affection, and for me it was the simple joy of our trio's togetherness.

By nine o'clock each night it was time to go home. Our mothers would telephone one another to arrange the pickups, and we girls would prepare to part ways. Bianca and I, though inseparable all evening, accepted the moment with grace. We would hug each other goodbye—tiny arms wrapped around each other in a ritual embrace that invariably caused a fond "aw" from whichever parent was watching. We knew tomorrow would reunite us, and that was enough. Marta, however, reacted differently. Nearly every time, she would burst into tears and protest the parting, despite the promise that we would all be together again the very next day. No amount of soothing words from the adults could console her in that moment of separation.

I often wondered, even then, why our parting hurt Marta so much more than it did Bianca or me. Was it simply an innate facet of her temperament, a heart born with an extra dose of longing, holding tighter to the moments she loved? Was her crying a plea for attention that she otherwise lacked, or was it the dread of returning to a house filled with tension and uncertainty instead of comfort and bedtime stories? Three girls, all of us the same age and raised in the same little neighborhood, sharing the same daily routines—yet we responded so differently to the simple event of saying goodnight. How could that be? The question fascinated me as a child and has lingered in my mind ever since. In a way, it was my first lesson in the secret complexity of human nature: even under similar circumstances, each child's emotional world is profoundly unique.

Even at eight years old, I tried my best to meet Marta in her feelings. I would pull her aside into a quiet corner of the living room, out of the adults' sight, and whisper to her that everything was alright. "It's fine, really," I would murmur, using the softest voice I could manage.

"We're just going to sleep and when morning comes, we'll be together again." I wanted to build a little bridge of words for her, one that could carry her safely over the long night until tomorrow reunited us. Sometimes my assurances calmed her for a moment; other times, nothing could stem her tears. Bianca and I learned to be patient with these outbursts, but I sometimes wondered if Marta's crying made us a little defensive, wary of getting too close to her emotions. Did her sadness push us away, even slightly? Or were her tears simply the visible cracks in a heart already stressed by sorrows that clearly lay beyond our understanding? The truth is, I will never know. In psychology—unlike in mathematics—causation and correlation blur like watercolors on paper. Two interpretations might both be true, or both false, while the real cause hides in layers we cannot see.

What I do know is that I felt an overwhelming desire to step into Marta's mind and make sense of her hurt. I wanted, more than anything, to see the world as she saw it and then translate reality back to her in a way that might bring her peace. The urge to understand someone's inner world so badly that I could help ease their pain never left me. Every "Marta" I have met since, every person whose emotions raged or sorrowed beyond my comprehension, has only stoked my curiosity more. It is as if that childhood farewell scene opened a door in me, leading to a lifelong quest to grasp the hidden workings of the heart. Don't we all?

Cruelty and Candor in the Playground

Childhood, as I soon discovered, is not all gentle curiosity and innocent tears. The schoolyard taught me about another side of human nature: the startling cruelty that children can inflict on one another. I was never the direct target of bullying, but I watched it unfold up close: classmates being humiliated for their differences, mocked for their quirks, or simply excluded from the group as though they were less than human. What shocked me even more was that I understood the bullies almost as much as I sympathized with their victims. I could see that there was a peculiar satisfaction, a pure desire (not a need, but a desire) in those bullies to diminish someone else, to establish themselves as powerful by making another feel small. It was an ugly impulse, yet disconcertingly familiar, as if I could recognize a shadow of it in my own heart.

Children can be unsparingly cruel; in fact, they are often the cruelest beings we encounter in life. A child has little concept of the damage words and exclusion can do, and so the blows they deal are startlingly blunt. Without guidance or correction, a child will quite readily unleash impulses of greed, jealousy, aggression, or spite. If no one intervenes to teach them kindness, empathy, and self-control, those impulses will solidify as habits. Cruel children, left unchecked, become cruel adults—or sometimes, adults who have learned to hide their cruelty beneath a veneer of social polish. The difference between most children and most adults is not that adults are purer in spirit, but simply that adults have learned, through education and discipline, to pretend. By adulthood we are practiced in the art of civility: we know how to smile and speak politely even when darker thoughts cross our minds. We respect the minimum boundaries that allow society to function; most of us do, at least. But that raw, unfiltered honesty of childhood—the kind that can manifest as brutal teasing on a playground—is still inside us. We are not better creatures than those children; we are merely better at concealing what they display openly.

The realization that the seeds of malice are present in all of us was both sobering and illuminating. It was tempting to believe that I, as a "good kid" who behaved and got good grades, was fundamentally different from the bully who stole lunch money or spread cruel rumors. Yet I could not deny that at times I, too, had felt a flash of anger, a sting of envy, or a mean thought that had no justification. The only difference was that something held me back from acting on those impulses, whereas the bullies I observed seemed to lack that restraint. What held me back, I suspect, were the lessons instilled by the adults in my life—my parents and teachers—who emphasized empathy and respect. The bullies, perhaps, had not absorbed those lessons, or had been taught entirely different ones by harsh experience. And so I saw clearly how crucial it was that children receive timely guidance on how to behave, how to master their fiercer impulses before those impulses mastered them.

Echoes of Human Darkness in History and Culture

It would be comforting to think that such cruelty is a childhood affliction, cured by the civilizing effects of growing up. But history provides far too many counterexamples. It was not always this way, that most adults behaved with a modicum of decency. Consider, for instance, a scene from the 16th century at the height of colonial conquest. Powerful men—respected leaders, kings and conquistadors—sent forth armies to invade foreign lands and subjugate entire peoples. These men, paragons of their societies, ordered and justified acts we now recognize as unspeakable atrocities. Entire villages turned to cinders; men, women, and children starved or forced into chains; vast populations deprived of freedom and dignity. No definition of "power," no flowery rhetoric of the time, could excuse what was in truth pure cruelty and greed. Today, we look back upon the colonizers with moral outrage. We condemn their deeds as crimes against humanity, wondering how those in the past could have been so blind and heartless.

We like to comfort ourselves with the belief that, had we lived in those times, we would have been different. We tell ourselves that we would never have committed such cruelties, never stayed silent while neighbors were enslaved or slaughtered. But here a troubling question must be asked: what makes us so sure we are fundamentally different from those men and women of the past? The capacity for darkness resides in the human soul across all eras. The same seeds of aggression, dominance, and fear that drove historical atrocities are still part of us today. We are fortunate to live in an age where certain brutal behaviors are outlawed and widely condemned—but the instinctual drive behind them has not vanished.

Just take a look at our popular culture for evidence. Consider the enduring popularity of a story like The Hunger Games. In that fictional universe, hapless youths are forced to kill one another in a televised tournament until a lone victor remains, all for the entertainment of a gleeful audience. When we read the book or watch the film, we naturally condemn the fictional citizens who cheer from the stands as the participants fight to the death. Yet we, the real-world audience, are positioned just like those citizens, watching violence as entertainment. We take in the spectacle of struggle and survival with popcorn in hand. We momentarily forget that, in essence, we are watching them watch people kill each other. It is a sobering meta-perspective: our enjoyment, however polished with moral commentary, still makes us participants in the same voyeurism of violence. This is not to say that enjoying a dark story makes us evil—far from it. But it reminds us that the line between us and the monsters we condemn is thinner than we would like to admit. Our fascination with fictional cruelty hints at something primal: a part of us that is drawn to darkness even as our conscious minds insist we stand on the side of the light.

Questioning the Reality of Goodness

By the time I was a teenager, I prided myself on being logical, rational, and firmly grounded in evidence. If something was ever wrong with my body, healthcare professionals could detect it with a blood test or an X-ray or a stethoscope. I believed the same about the mind: that clear facts would lead to clear conclusions. This almost naïve faith in facts made it all more disorienting when I found myself facing struggles that facts and logic alone could not resolve.

In my late teens and early twenties, I began to experience the first shadows of mental anguish—bouts of sadness and anxiety that I could not explain for sure why. At first, I questioned whether these struggles were even real. Was I actually depressed, or was I somehow inventing symptoms in my head, and sabotaging my own peace? I interrogated the concept of depression relentlessly, pulling it apart in my mind. Was depression exactly what the textbooks described—an illness with specific criteria? Or was it something broader and more elusive, a spiritual vacuum, a collapse of meaning? Could it sometimes be less than a disease, more a passing storm than a chronic climate? I even caught myself doubting others who claimed to suffer. A quiet, troubling whisper took root in my mind: What if some of these people are lying, even to themselves? How can we ever truly prove, or measure, the pain of a mind?

These doubts grew even sharper after I moved from Brazil to the United States. Back in my hometown of Goiânia, I had been one of the top students in my school, perhaps the top student in the entire year. I was hungry for knowledge, driven each day by an almost reflexive ambition to excel. When I arrived in New York, I found myself in a place where all the conditions for success were finally in place—an esteemed university, a world of opportunities spread out before me. By all logic, I should have been thriving. And yet, to my great confusion, the spark within me began to fade. The light in my eyes lost some of its shine and I could not explain why. I would wake in the mornings not with excitement but with a heavy cloud of fatigue and somewhat lazyness. I wondered if it was just the weight of adapting to a new world—new language, new culture, far from home—or if it was something more intimate and fundamental. I found myself asking the most basic question: Why get out of bed today? And a quiet truth emerged in response: because, at the bottom of everything, I wanted to feel that I mattered to someone. I began to see that beyond ambition or adventure, there was a more essential human need at play—the need to be seen, to be remembered, to be loved. Love, I realized, was what lends energy to our days, what keeps us moving forward even when logic gives us no grand answer. Without feeling connected to others—without love in some form— achievements and opportunities felt strangely hollow. And it turned out that I ended up in a city in which none of the people I loved (at that point) was. This realization humbled me deeply. It hinted that underneath all our rational plans and proud ideals, we remain driven by the same emotional currents that guided us as children: the need to feel safe, valued, and loved for who we are.

Goodness, Naïveté, and the Seeds of Resentment

Coming to terms with my own darkness and needs made me reflect on the people around me—especially those I had always considered truly "good." Over the years I have been fortunate to know many kind-hearted souls. By good, I mean people whose empathy outweighs their envy, who offer help without calculating what they might get in return, who genuinely wish to make the world better even if no one thanks them. I admired such people deeply. For a long time, I even believed that their goodness was so pure that they might be incapable of harmful intent. I caught myself thinking that maybe truly good people never felt angry at all—at least not in the vindictive, simmering way that leads to cruelty. It was a comforting thought, but one that life experience would later unravel.

I began to notice something subtle: those very kind and gentle people, the ones who never seemed upset on the surface, sometimes carried a quiet undercurrent of resentment. Outwardly, they never raised their voice, never spoke an unkind word. But small injustices and unspoken slights were accumulating in them like steam in a sealed kettle. Because they saw themselves as kind (or needed to see themselves that way) they suppressed their anger at others for far too long. Eventually, inevitably, there would come a moment when the pressure became too great. Then the explosion would come, seemingly out of nowhere, and often directed at someone who had little to do with the original hurt. I saw a gentle friend snap in fury over a trivial inconvenience; I saw a compassionate colleague break into sobs of rage over an innocent remark. It was as if all the denied anger, stored up for years, had finally found a weak spot in the dam. And here was the most startling revelation: this pattern of restraint and outburst did not arise suddenly in adulthood—it had roots tracing back to childhood. The shift from quiet goodness to misplaced fury was not a new skill learned later in life; it was the delayed consequence of habits formed when they were young. A child who is taught to "be nice" at all costs, to never express anger, may grow into an adult who knows no healthy way to cope when they are wronged.

This realization forced me to confront a myth I had unwittingly believed: the myth that human souls start out pure and are only corrupted by the world. I came to see that the human soul is not inherently innocent or pure white—it carries every color, every shade from the very beginning. Watch any group of children at play and you will see it: the capacity for love and joy, certainly, but also flashes of greed, envy, dominance, and deceit. Yes, how a child is raised will encourage some traits and discourage others, but every child contains the seeds of both good and evil. Bullying behavior in a child can indeed be exacerbated by a cruel or neglectful home—but it also arises unprompted from the child's own untamed temperament. And if that temperament—the fierce, aggressive streak in a naturally dominant child, or the anxious, sensitive streak in a naturally timid one—is ignored or mishandled by adults, the child's way of coping with the world solidifies in whatever shape it has learned, for better or for worse. In short, our nature has a say in who we become, as surely as nurture does.

I had to admit to myself that I, too, carried a share of those darker instincts. For years I maintained a self-image of being a "good person" because I was polite and helpful, even as I privately wrestled with darker thoughts—flashes of anger, selfishness, even cruelty—that I dared not show. I worried that these thoughts made me a fraud, unworthy of the goodness I tried to embody. But that illusion of personal purity eventually crumbled. I came to learn that even the kindest, gentlest people you will ever meet have their wicked thoughts. The difference is that they recognize them (or fail to), and choose not to act on them (or eventually lose control). When I learned this (truly learned it, not just as a saying but as a lived truth) it was a relief. I finally felt I belonged to the human family, with all its flaws. I was not a solitary monster hiding among saints; I was simply human, like everyone else, capable of both kindness and cruelty.

If naive innocence is fragile, untested goodness is downright dangerous. A person convinced of their own pure goodness can be shockingly unprepared for the reality of temptation and malice, in themselves or in others. In my case, I realized my idealized view of "good people" had made me gullible. I took others at face value, assuming the version of themselves they presented publicly was the whole truth. This was no different, I later understood, from falling for the curated perfection of an Instagram feed or a glossy TikTok clip... Only I had fallen for it in real life interactions. I believed the masks that people wear in polite society, because I wanted to believe in the purity they projected. When evidence to the contrary finally broke through my denial, I felt disillusioned, even betrayed. But ultimately, shedding that naive belief was liberating. It allowed me to replace judgment with compassion: to understand that everyone has an inner life more complex than they show, that even those who seem to "have it all together" struggle with ugly thoughts and inner demons. And if we are all struggling in this way, who am I to judge anyone harshly? My friends sometimes remark that I can be shockingly free of judgment, even when someone admits to a terrible thought or mistake. It isn't that I approve of wrongdoing, but I just see in their confession the same humanity that lives in me. We are all made of the same clay, light and dark swirled together. The mind is an extraordinary landscape: vast in its capacity for love and hate, creativity and destruction. I would be lying to deny that complexity, in them or in myself.

The Discipline of Mastering Our Impulses

Dark thoughts and fierce impulses arise within us unbidden: fantasies of betrayal or revenge, flashes of anger and aggression, even images of destruction or perversion that seem to have no place in our peaceable daily lives. One of the great marvels of being human, I have come to believe, is not that we have such thoughts; it is that we have the capacity to choose what to do about them. The mark of a mature soul is not pristine thinking, but the ability to control our worst impulses and channel them, when possible, toward something good. In a sense, our true strength lies in our self-mastery. Life will continually present us with lessons in this form: situations that provoke our anger or fear, moments when our most primitive reactions surge up. Each time, we face a choice. We can lash out or succumb, letting those impulses dictate our behavior; or we can take a step back, recognize the impulse for what it is, and decide whether acting on it will serve any good. This discipline of acknowledging without obeying our darker emotions is one of the hardest things to learn, but it is perhaps the most important lesson of growing up. Ironically, it is a lesson we often drill into children, "Control yourself!" "Use your words!" and yet as adults we sometimes fail to practice it ourselves, opting instead for denial or repression. I learned that real courage and character involve facing the roaring ocean inside us, not denying it exists, and steering our ship through its waves with both firmness and compassion.

Interestingly, the roots of both our darkest aggressions and our brightest virtues are often one and the same. The very capacity for anger and aggression, which can manifest as cruelty, is also the source of courage and bravery when properly harnessed. A child with a strong will and fiery temper might, under poor guidance, become a bully or an outcast. But under wise guidance, that same child might grow into a bold truth-teller, a leader unafraid to stand against injustice. The difference lies not in extinguishing the flame, but in teaching how it can light a hearth instead of a forest fire. This is why the environment in which we are raised matters so deeply. The task of parents, and of any society entrusted with the care of its young, is not to pretend that children are angelic beings of pure goodness. It is to recognize the full spectrum within them (the potential for good and the potential for evil) and to help them understand and govern that inner diversity. Historically, different cultures have approached this task in various ways. For generations, many parents were stricter with sons and more protective of daughters, believing this prepared boys for a harsh world and kept girls safe from it. In our modern era, we are rethinking those patterns. I have observed, for example, that many contemporary mothers (with the best of intentions) have become exceedingly gentle and indulgent with their sons, shielding them from all distress; perhaps a reaction to the call for a kinder, less aggressively "masculine" man. Yet this very softness can backfire, leaving those boys ill-equipped to handle the real conflicts and challenges of adult life. On the other hand, girls today are encouraged to be strong and independent, which is a wonderful progress, though it sometimes comes paired with a narrative of perpetual victimhood ("we are not truly free or safe"), even in societies where women enjoy more freedom and opportunity than ever before in history.

The paradoxes of modern parenting and social conditioning are complex. The overprotectiveness many of us experienced as children, born from our parents' fear of the world's cruelty, has in some cases bred a generation of cautious, even cowardly adults. Having faced little hardship or having had every conflict mediated for them, many grown men and women find themselves unequipped to assert themselves or to cope with the normal frictions of life. I have met far too many adults whose timidity and passivity trace back to a childhood where any risk was smothered by a hovering parent. And ironically, much of this overprotection stems from a place of love: parents who once endured bullying or trauma often vow that their children should never suffer the same, and in shielding them excessively, they unintentionally also shield them from growth.

Children, in their own right, wield surprising social power over each other—through charm, intimidation, or sheer obstinacy, even a young child can bend a whole family's patterns around their will. Any parent who has navigated the moods of a toddler or the dramas of a teenager knows this well. Thus, raising a child into a balanced adult is a dance of constant adjustment and wisdom. You must neither crush the child's spirit nor let the child rule like a tyrant. It requires recognizing that the roots of anger and aggression are the very same roots from which empathy and courage spring forth. A child who is never allowed to express anger may never learn to defend themselves or others when it truly matters; a child who is never taught to rein in their impulses may trample over others' rights without remorse.

Raising a Resilient Child

If I ever have a child of my own—be it a son or a daughter of any temperament—my deepest wish would be to see them grow as early as possible into a functional, whole person, comfortable in their own skin. To that end, I would strive to create an environment that inoculates them against the cruelty of the world; not by hiding them away, but by making home a place of unconditional acceptance and strength. If I feared my child might face bullying outside, I would make absolutely certain that no bullying or belittlement took place under my own roof. Home should be the one place where a child feels 100% accepted for who they are. No ridicule for their quirks, no pressure to be someone they are not, just to appease the preferences of others outside the family. Within the walls of our home, they would know that they are loved without condition. From that secure base, I would also teach them how to defend themselves in the wider world—not to seek fights or harbor a perpetual victim mindset, but to stand up calmly for their own dignity.

Too often, I have seen parents use the excuse of "preparing the child for the cruel outside world" as a thin veil over their own prejudices or unreasonable expectations of their kids. A father ashamed of a son's gentle demeanor, a mother uneasy about a daughter's boldness—sometimes the parent will claim they are worried how others will treat the child, when in truth it is they who cannot accept some aspect of their own offspring. This is a cruel illusion that can quietly wreck a child's sense of self. A child who grows up feeling that their parents are embarrassed by them, or wish them to be someone else, carries a heavy burden of shame. That shame can trail them into adulthood like a shadow, undermining their confidence at every step. On the other hand, a child who hears from the start (through both words and actions) that they are valued, supported, and believed in, gains a kind of armor against the world's inevitable slings and arrows. The world may still hurt them, yes, but the wounds will not fester as deeply because the child knows, in their heart, "I am worthy and I am loved." What we say to our children becomes the voice they carry inside them for life. This truth has made me more mindful of how I speak not only to children, but to the child that still lives in each of us. We all have an "inner child," formed from the echoes of what our caretakers once told us about ourselves. If that inner child learns only fear and criticism, part of growing up is learning to re-parent ourselves: to provide the encouragement or discipline we may not have received, and to undo the cruel illusions we may have accepted about our own worth.

But here comes the most important part: while love and acceptance are crucial, structure and discipline form the other side of the coin for healthy growth. A family that provides affection but no guidance can leave a child just as lost as one that provides criticism without love. Children test boundaries not because they want to break them, but often to discover that the boundaries are there, that the world has structure, that some choices lead to harm and others to harmony. Telling a child "no" when necessary, grounding them for misbehavior, insisting they take responsibility for their actions—these are also acts of love, though they are difficult and sometimes heart-wrenching in the moment. It is far easier for a parent to yield, to say "yes" just to avoid a tantrum, to tidy up the mess rather than make the child clean it, to excuse bad behavior as "just being a kid." But easy love, love without facing the child's temporary anger or tears, often creates a fragile adult. If we do not help a child confront the consequences of their actions, we set them up for a cruel collision with reality later on. In essence, the surest way to raise a resilient child is to neither crush their spirit nor coddle it. Guide them, but let them feel the wind and occasionally the fall; embrace them, but let them wrestle with their own frustrations and find their way through. They will thank you later with a confidence that rests quietly in their bones. Finally, let us address a curious contradiction of our times. We live in an era where, arguably, women and men in many societies enjoy more legal rights and freedoms than at any previous point in human history. A woman today (in much of the world) may choose whether or not to marry, to pursue any education or career that calls to her, to vote and voice her opinions, to lead a company or a country, or to devote herself to raising children—or indeed, to do both. She can decide that motherhood is central to her happiness, or decide to live happily without children. These choices, which we now take almost for granted, were dreams scarcely imaginable for our great-grandmothers.

In this sense, we are the freest generation of women ever to walk the Earth. And yet, I often hear an odd refrain from some corners: "We are not free." It is usually spoken as a political slogan or a rallying cry. I sometimes worry that we have become so focused on what we lack that we fail to cherish what we have. Likewise, at the very same time that some declare women to be perpetually oppressed, I see many of these same voices raising their sons with a kind of unchecked indulgence, as if oblivious to the quiet irony. A mother who proclaims "No man will ever have authority over me!" may, in the next breath, bend over backwards to satisfy every whim of her little boy—thus granting him, at age five, more authority over her daily life than any grown man could ever hope to wield.

These ironies are not condemnations but illustrations of how complicated the human psyche can be. We rebel against one imbalance only to slide into another. The rise of a more conscientious femininity in society coincided, in many households, with a sort of new princely status for boys, whose mothers and fathers, eager to correct the past, perhaps overcorrected in the present. The result, as I see it, has been confusion all around: daughters taught to fear the very vulnerability that can give life depth and meaning, and sons taught to expect a level of adoration from the world that no adult man will ever receive.

A Time to Feel, a Time to Reign Ourselves In

All of these threads — from playground cruelties to the indulgences and paradoxes of modern parenting — tie back to a central truth about human nature. It is in our nature to feel everything: to be angry, envious, joyful, courageous, creative, loving, and yes, at times cruel. Every emotion, from the noblest to the most shameful, rises up in us unbidden, just as storms rise in the atmosphere. These emotions and impulses are not evil in themselves; they are simply part of us, as natural as the weather. In childhood, with its bursts of anger and sudden tenderness, we see this truth plainly. Children feel intensely and show it. In a healthy upbringing, they are taught gradually how to weather those inner storms: how to let the rain of emotion fall without flooding the whole landscape. We teach them not to hit when they're angry, not to grab in their greed, not to collapse in despair when they lose. We teach them, in essence, how to feel everything, yet not be ruled by those feelings.

Yet somewhere along the passage into adulthood, many of us betray this very lesson. We begin to treat our own inner life as though it were an unwelcome intruder to be silenced or locked away. The child is taught to master their tempests, but the grown man or woman chooses instead the easier habit of repression. Rather than acknowledging "I am angry" or "I am hurt" and then working through it as we might instruct a child to do, we simply shove the feeling down and pretend it doesn't exist. We have, in a sense, lost faith in our ability to guide ourselves, even though we managed to guide our children. The result is a paradox, even a tragedy: the very people who once helped a child find balance become adults who have lost their own.

From that failure of emotional courage, the distorted landscape of our present age has emerged. It is an era in which men and women, unable to live with the simple candor of their youth, seek refuge in extremes. Some chase excess by throwing themselves into work, or drink, or material accumulation to distract from the emotions they refuse to confront. Others cling to the hollow prestige of outward appearances, crafting perfect lives on social media while privately drowning in loneliness. Many simply drift, neither truly feeling nor truly living, caught in endless distractions because silence and self-honesty have become too foreign and frightening. Wouldn't it be much easier had we chosen to learn how to express our feelings?

But it need not remain this way. If there is a truth this first chapter hopes to convey, it is that to be human is not to be pure, but to be whole. Wholeness means embracing every part of ourselves—the light and the dark, the child and the adult, the rage and the love—and learning to integrate them. The journey ahead, through the coming chapters, will explore how we might reclaim that wholeness. It will ask why we have strayed so far from the wisdom we try to impart to our children, and how we might find our way back. After all, the child we each once were is still within us, waiting with open eyes and honest emotions. It falls to us now, as adults, to take that child by the hand

and finally say, "Come, show me how to feel again and together we will learn how to be strong."

Childhood, with its bursts of anger and sudden tenderness, teaches us that to be human is to be whole. Yet somewhere along the passage into adulthood, we began to treat our own inner life as though it were an intruder to be silenced. We reached a paradox: the very ones who once guided the child toward balance became adults who could no longer guide themselves. From that failure emerged the distorted landscape of the present age — an era where men and women, unable to live by the simple candor of their youth, surrendered themselves to the endless pursuits of excess, distraction, and the hollow prestige of appearances.

CHAPTER 2

The Modern Mind in Crisis

There are mornings in every great city when one can witness a spectacle both ordinary and unsettling. Step into the subway at rush hour and you will see hundreds of faces illuminated by the pale glow of screens. Eyes fix upon images that vanish as quickly as they appear, fingers move with restless repetition, and the entire crowd seems suspended in a half-silence – not quite present, not quite absent, adrift between distraction and fatigue. Here, in this anonymous crowd, lies a portrait of our age: a civilization abundant in resources yet impoverished in spirit, busier than ever yet unable to say why they are in a hurry at all.

For the modern citizen, life is a paradox. We possess comforts and securities that not even kings of earlier centuries could scarcely have imagined. Hunger and plague no longer haunt our nights; wars are fewer, luxuries more accessible, knowledge available at the tap of a finger. And yet, amid these triumphs, despair has not retreated. Anxiety disorders rise each year, depression spreads like a silent fog, suicidality reaches the young before they have scarcely begun to live, and addictions of all kinds have woven themselves into the very fabric of daily existence. By almost every external measure, life has improved; by the internal measure of the soul, it has withered.

It is common to believe that life would be easier if people could freely express their opinions. I take it further: life would not only be easier, but it would also be resolved. Think of the Uber driver who, after fifteen minutes of conversation, is convinced that if the country were run according to his ideas, it would be in a far better place. The history student who insists her professor is incompetent believes that if she taught the class, her students would flourish. The wealthy employer who could transform the life of a homeless man simply by donating ten percent of his salary—and yet does not. The friend who could have achieved so much by now if only he stopped smoking. And of course, there is you, convinced that without your influence, someone you care about would never break free from the spiral they are trapped in.

On paper, these thoughts sound naive, almost simplistic. Yet this is how most people operate without even realizing it. They act with the conviction that they hold the one and only truth. The problem is that certainty without depth breeds division rather than solutions. When people speak from a place of shallow knowledge, their argument begins to crumble after the third sentence. They cannot sustain their own conviction under examination.

I was like this for a long time. This book that you are reading right now? It has been in my head for the past 5 years, but I only published it now. I grew up with compliments all around me about how smart and proactive I am, but my ideas were just ideas until I finally decided to take action. How many businesses have you thought about and never concluded?

Here is where the challenge lies. If you want to express your opinions, then own them completely. Be prepared to defend them not with bluster, but with clarity. To own an opinion is to take responsibility for it, to accept that it will be questioned, and to stand by it with the same strength you had when you first voiced it. Choosing silence is not neutral—it aligns you with the very passivity you might condemn in others. If you are strong enough to stand by your thoughts, you must also be strong enough to articulate them.

This is what the modern world lacks. We are overflowing with strong opinions, but starved of action. Cowardice has become a defining feature of our time, where the loudest voices are filtered through the safe distance of social media rather than spoken face to face. And in my view, there is something even more dangerous in this: the weakest people, whether in body, mind, or will, are often the quickest to become dangerous. The absence of expression is a form of expression—it speaks loudly in its own way.

Consider the man who refuses to protect his wife on the grounds that she is strong and independent. He is far more dangerous than the man who steps forward to protect her. Why? Because in denying the instinct to act, he suppresses something fundamental to his nature, replacing it with an idea that does not align with his own emotions or biology. Suppressed instincts breed resentment, and resentment often seeks an outlet. Too often, that outlet is an act of cowardice disguised as restraint, a silent bitterness that hides behind screens or polite detachment.

Cowardice is not the only problem. The space left behind by those who lack courage becomes fertile ground for others to dominate. The few who do speak begin to shape the narrative, unchecked, while the silent majority becomes increasingly vulnerable to manipulation. Power, then, rests in the hands of an ever-shrinking circle. Think about it: how many musicians are truly relevant? How many authors are truly read? There are brilliant voices that never leave the page, minds that never share their insights because their owners remain silent. This is how oppression takes root—not always through force, but through the self-imposed silence of those who could have spoken.

This is the crisis of the modern mind: a ceaseless motion that mistakes accumulation for meaning, and a restless anxiety that confuses noise for vitality. But the consequences of such a life are not borne in the abstract alone. They carve themselves into the very fabric of the brain. Every hurried indulgence, every unexamined desire, every abandonment of purpose leaves its trace upon the nervous system, as if culture itself were etching its disquiet into biology. What once seemed merely a moral disorientation now reveals itself as a physiological wound: the sick brain, formed at the crossroads where society's illusions meet the vulnerabilities of human nature. To understand this affliction, we must descend further — from the surface of cultural despair into the hidden mechanisms of the mind, where chemistry and memory conspire to shape disorder.

How did we arrive here? It is tempting to answer with statistics, with the language of economics and epidemiology. We might say that globalization fractured our sense of home, that technology compressed time into an unending now, that consumerism promised happiness only to deliver emptiness. All these explanations contain truth, but none is sufficient. The real story is more intimate, more subtle. It is the story of a man who, despite being surrounded by wonders, finds his mornings unbearable; of a woman whose life is secure yet whose nights are consumed by loneliness; of a generation that, though liberated from the burdens of history, finds itself paralyzed before the future. It is not hunger or poverty that undoes them, but a crisis at once moral, psychological, and biological: a crisis lodged in the very workings of the brain.

What we face today is not a new plague, though its reach is epidemic. It is a slow erosion of meaning, responsibility, and intimacy: the very elements that once gave life its texture. When purpose weakens, emotions lose their anchor; when responsibility is abandoned, will collapses into cowardice; when intimacy falters, even love becomes fragile. The individual thus adrift seeks substitutes: a drink at night, a pill in the morning, the glowing distraction of a screen at every spare moment. These substitutes promise relief, but they also tighten the chains of dependency. Neuroscience explains that dopamine systems designed to reward discovery and effort are now hijacked by drugs and algorithms, leaving the mind restless, hungry, and perpetually dissatisfied. What begins as a choice for ease becomes a trap of compulsion, and what begins as a pursuit of comfort ends as an illness of despair.

Yet it would be a mistake to treat these difficulties merely as medical curiosities, to be solved by prescriptions alone. They are not accidents of chemistry but symptoms of a deeper malaise. A society that celebrates shortcuts, that elevates safety above courage, that distracts rather than dreams, creates the conditions in which the brain itself grows sick. The anxious individual is not a statistical outlier; he is the emblem of a culture that has lost its balance between order and chaos. The depressive is not a tragic anomaly; she is the mirror of a world that whispers endlessly that nothing truly matters. Even suicide, the most devastating of outcomes, is not merely a private calamity; it is the logical terminus of a society that teaches its children to repress their emotions, to consume their days in distraction, and to live without a horizon of meaning.

In earlier centuries, suffering at least bore the dignity of necessity. Hunger came because crops failed, plague because sanitation was primitive, war because empires clashed. Today, suffering arrives stripped of such explanations. We suffer not from too little, but from too much; not from famine, but from excess; not from silence, but from noise. The human mind, evolved for endurance and scarcity, now confronts abundance without compass, speed without destination, connection without intimacy. It is no wonder, then, that it falters. For the brain, like the soul, requires structure, purpose, and limits — and without them, it collapses under the weight of its own freedom.

One sees the evidence everywhere. The child who cannot imagine a future beyond the next video. The young professional who, despite security and success, feels an unnamed hollowness gnaw at his days. The couple who lie side by side in bed, each illuminated by a separate screen, their intimacy slowly dissolving into pixels. The elderly parent who watches his grown children, prosperous but estranged, and wonders what became of the bonds that once held families together. These are not isolated misfortunes; they are chapters in a single story, the story of a civilization that has gained the world and yet risks losing its soul.

This book speaks of the sick brain, but we must understand from the outset: the brain does not fall ill in isolation. It becomes sick because society itself has shifted in ways that press upon the nervous system with relentless force. The erosion of meaning, the abdication of responsibility, the cult of shortcuts, the worship of comfort, the death of dreaming, and the collapse of intimacy — these are not abstract moral defects but living conditions that inscribe themselves into neurons, synapses, and circuits. They create an environment in which anxiety flourishes, depression deepens, and addiction becomes not the exception but the norm.

Thus, to understand the modern mind in crisis, we must look both outward and inward: outward, to the cultural currents that have reshaped our lives; inward, to the biological consequences that emerge when those currents overwhelm the brain. Only by tracing this double movement can we begin to see why despair has become the companion of abundance, why anxiety flourishes in the midst of freedom, and why, in an age of unprecedented connection, loneliness remains one of the most common afflictions.

The chapters that follow will unfold this story. We will examine the seven great problems of our time, each a thread in the tangled fabric of our malaise. We will see how they distort our relationships, sap our self-esteem, cloud our moods, and ultimately bend the brain itself toward illness. And we will glimpse, too, the possibility of healing — for to name a disease is the first step toward its cure. But before we search for remedies, we must confront the diagnosis. We must dare to look at the civilization we have built, at once dazzling and despairing, and admit: we are adrift.

When Friedrich Nietzsche declared, more than a century ago, that "God is dead," he was not celebrating a victory but announcing a calamity. He foresaw that the decline of transcendence, of shared myth and sacred order, would leave man staggering beneath the weight of freedom. What he could not yet know was how prophetic his warning would become. For in our time, the erosion of meaning is not the concern of philosophers alone; it is the silent epidemic shaping millions of lives.

To live without meaning is to live without orientation. The human brain, with its restless search for patterns and goals, is not content with survival alone; it demands a story, a reason to endure suffering, a horizon toward which effort is directed. Without such a horizon, pain becomes unbearable and pleasure becomes empty. Neuroscience confirms this ancient truth: the dopaminergic pathways of the brain are not activated merely by reward but by the anticipation of reward, by the belief that present struggle serves a future purpose. Strip life of that purpose and the brain itself falters; motivation weakens, resilience declines, despair grows.

In earlier centuries, meaning was not optional. Religion, ritual, and tradition provided scaffolding for existence. Even the poorest peasant, laboring in the fields, understood himself as part of a story larger than his hunger: he worked not only for bread but for God, for family, for community. That scaffolding has eroded. Religion has lost its authority for many; traditions have withered in the face of modern individualism; families scatter under the demands of mobility and ambition. What remains is the naked self, alone before the void, told that he is free to invent his own purpose. Freedom, without a compass, becomes paralysis.

It is no coincidence that the loss of meaning coincides with rising anxiety. For anxiety is not only fear of the unknown; it is the dread of navigating a world with no reliable map. If life is nothing more than a sequence of appetites and distractions, then every failure looms catastrophic, every setback threatens annihilation. A man without meaning cannot endure misfortune; he interprets suffering not as part of a story but as proof of absurdity. Thus, he oscillates between frantic pursuit of pleasure and the crushing suspicion that none of it matters.

Consider the modern professional who, by all outward measures, has succeeded. He is educated, employed, perhaps even affluent. Yet when he rises each morning, he feels the weight of futility pressing against his chest. His days are consumed by tasks whose purpose he cannot articulate; his evenings dissolve into the glow of a screen. He wonders, silently and with shame, whether this is all life offers. His despair is not born of poverty but of purposelessness. It is not that he suffers too much; it is that his suffering appears to serve no end. Such lives are increasingly common. We see them in students who, despite unprecedented opportunity, collapse under stress and self-doubt; in parents who, despite comfort and security, feel estranged from their children; in entire societies where, amid luxury, loneliness festers. The question "why live?" once answered by faith, duty, or communal bonds, now falls heavily upon the solitary individual. And when he cannot answer, the consequences are grave. Depression, at its core, is a disease of meaning: it whispers that nothing matters, that no effort will alter the outcome, that existence itself is futile. Suicide, its most tragic expression, is not chosen because life is unbearable in fact, but because life is unbearable when believed to be without meaning.

In the absence of purpose, substitutes proliferate. Consumer culture offers the promise of happiness through acquisition: the new phone, the larger home, the exotic vacation. Yet the satisfaction fades quickly, leaving behind only the need for more. Social media offers the illusion of significance through visibility: likes, followers, recognition by strangers. But this too is fleeting, and worse, it binds self-worth to the fickle approval of others. Drugs and alcohol offer relief from the gnawing emptiness, but only by deepening dependence. Each substitute masks despair for a moment, only to intensify it in the long run.

The collapse of meaning does not remain confined to the solitary mind; it corrodes relationships. Love demands a sense of future — the promise that two lives intertwined will build something larger than either alone. But when the future appears hollow, intimacy dissolves into transaction. Sexuality, stripped of meaning, becomes a fleeting exchange, incapable of offering the stability the psyche craves. Self-esteem, too, falters in the absence of purpose. For one's worth cannot be measured solely by appearance or income; it requires the deeper conviction that one's existence serves a goal beyond the self. Without that conviction, even success tastes of ash.

We deceive ourselves if we imagine that the collapse of meaning is a problem for philosophers alone. It is a clinical reality. The rising tide of anxiety, depression, and suicidality is not merely a medical mystery but the biological echo of a society that has lost its narrative. When the individual is told to invent his own purpose, but given no tools to do so, the brain's motivational systems falter. Dopamine circuits, deprived of enduring goals, fall prey to short-term distractions and addictions. The result is not freedom but enslavement — enslavement to substances, to screens, to restless consumption.

Yet the hunger for meaning persists. Even those who claim life is absurd betray, in their actions, a longing for more. Why else seek recognition, love, or achievement, if not to escape the insignificance they confess? The paradox of our time is that we live as though nothing matters while behaving as though everything does. We deny transcendence yet crave it; we dismiss responsibility yet suffer without it; we drown ourselves in distraction yet complain of boredom. This tension, unresolved, breeds the very illnesses we lament.

What is at stake is not merely the individual psyche but civilization itself. A culture that cannot provide meaning will not sustain itself. Its citizens, restless and despairing, will turn to extremes: addiction, escapism, nihilism, or even violence. History shows this pattern: when societies lose their guiding myths, they fracture, and into the vacuum rush ideologies that promise purpose, however destructive. In this sense, the crisis of meaning is not only personal but political, not only biological but civilizational.

To rebuild meaning is no simple task. It requires not a return to superstition but a rediscovery of responsibility, community, and love. It requires individuals to confront suffering not as an error but as the very soil of growth. It requires us to dream again, to imagine futures worth striving toward. For without such dreams, life collapses into monotony, and monotony into despair. Meaning cannot be handed down like a commodity; it must be lived. But society can at least provide the conditions for its pursuit: spaces of silence, traditions of purpose, relationships of trust.

The collapse of meaning is the first wound of the modern mind, and perhaps the deepest. It is the silent undertow that drags countless lives toward anxiety, depression, and addiction. Unless we confront it, all other remedies are palliative. For no pill, no possession, no fleeting pleasure can replace the quiet conviction that life, in its hardship and in its joy, is worth living. And it is this conviction, fragile yet indispensable, that we have allowed to slip from our grasp.

If the loss of meaning is the silent undertow of our age, then the abdication of responsibility is its most visible tide. Responsibility is what binds the chaos of existence into order; it is the weight that gives shape to a life. To be responsible is to recognize that one's actions matter, that the smallest decision ripples outward into family, community, and society. It is to say: "I will carry this burden, even if I did not choose it, even if I cannot master it fully, for in carrying it I become more than myself." And yet, in our time, responsibility has been recast as a burden to be avoided, a nuisance that interferes with the pursuit of comfort and autonomy. What earlier generations regarded as the foundation of dignity, we increasingly treat as an obstacle to personal freedom.

The irony, of course, is that the flight from responsibility does not liberate but enslaves. Cowardice, though it pretends to make life lighter, leaves the soul hollow. A man who refuses to take responsibility for his work, his family, or even his own emotions, is not free; he is at the mercy of circumstance. He becomes like a leaf carried by the wind, convinced he is floating by choice, when in truth he has surrendered all direction. Cowardice whispers: "You deserve ease. You are entitled to relief. You need not endure hardship." And yet the fruit of that whisper is not peace but fragility, a will unprepared for adversity, a spirit untrained for life's inevitable storms.

This phenomenon is not merely moral but psychological. The prefrontal cortex, that region of the brain responsible for decision-making and impulse control, develops and strengthens through the assumption of responsibility. Children who are taught to complete tasks, to resist impulses, to care for others, build neural pathways that equip them for adult resilience. But adults who habitually avoid responsibility — who drown their obligations in excuses or outsource them to others — weaken the very circuits that once gave them strength. Avoidance does not simply leave duties undone; it reshapes the brain into an organ of passivity. Neuroscience here converges with philosophy: to live without responsibility is to unmake oneself. This abdication has subtle forms. In the workplace, it appears as the refusal to own mistakes, the endless shifting of blame from one colleague to another. In the family, it manifests as parents who outsource the raising of children to screens and institutions, claiming exhaustion while forgetting that love is always exhausting. In society, it surfaces as citizens who demand rights yet shirk duties, who cry out for justice but recoil when asked to act justly themselves. Each instance may appear trivial, but taken together, they form a culture where cowardice masquerades as normalcy.

The consequences are profound. Cowardice breeds resentment, for a man who refuses responsibility still suffers, and in suffering he looks for someone to blame. When no one else can be found, he turns against himself, collapsing into anxiety or despair. Alternatively, he directs his resentment outward, into grievance, outrage, or even violence. Without responsibility, life's hardships become intolerable, for they seem undeserved; and without the discipline of responsibility, even life's pleasures become unsteady, for they lack the anchor of accomplishment. Thus cowardice robs man not only of dignity but of stability.

Consider the young adult who, upon leaving home, is told that life should be easy, that his happiness is the responsibility of institutions, parents, or partners. Each obstacle he encounters appears as an injustice, each demand as oppression. Rather than grow resilient, he grows brittle; rather than face his suffering, he seeks escape. Soon he discovers that chemical substances and digital distractions offer temporary relief, and so he surrenders to them. But these substitutes cannot carry responsibility for him; they only deepen his incapacity to carry it himself. Thus cowardice becomes addiction, and addiction becomes despair.

History reminds us that civilizations rise on the shoulders of those who accept responsibility and fall when that virtue declines. The builders of cathedrals, the explorers of oceans, the defenders of liberty — all bore burdens they could have avoided, yet chose not to. They knew that freedom without duty is chaos, and that dignity without sacrifice is an illusion. Our era, by contrast, often celebrates the opposite. The idol of personal freedom is raised so high that responsibility appears almost offensive, a relic of a harsher past. Yet the result is not liberation but collapse, for a society of individuals unwilling to bear burdens is a society unable to endure.

At its heart, cowardice is not the absence of fear but the refusal to confront it. Every human life is marked by fear: fear of failure, of rejection, of loss, of suffering. To take responsibility is to face those fears and to say: "Though I am afraid, I will act." To refuse responsibility is to let fear dictate existence. The coward convinces himself that he avoids responsibility because life is unjust, because others are corrupt, because the burden is too heavy. But beneath these justifications lies a single truth: he has allowed fear to govern him. And a life governed by fear cannot be free.

The consequences of cowardice penetrate even the most intimate realms of human life. Love itself requires responsibility — the courage to remain faithful, the patience to endure difficulty, the discipline to nurture another's growth. Yet when cowardice rules, love collapses into selfishness. Relationships become fragile, partnerships dissolve at the first sign of hardship, intimacy is replaced by convenience. A man who will not carry responsibility for himself cannot carry it for another, and thus his capacity for love atrophies. What remains is not union but transaction, not intimacy but escape. In this way, cowardice does not only weaken society; it impoverishes the heart.

It is tempting to imagine that responsibility can be indefinitely postponed, that someone else will always carry the burden. But the reality is harsher. Responsibilities abandoned do not vanish; they accumulate. They appear later in the form of broken families, fractured communities, or personal collapse. The man who refuses to care for his health will later be enslaved by illness; the parent who avoids disciplining his child will later face rebellion; the citizen who refuses civic duty will later inherit corruption. Responsibility ignored is responsibility compounded. The coward pays eventually, and often with interest.

If there is any hope, it lies in remembering that responsibility, though heavy, is also liberating. To take responsibility is to claim agency, to affirm that one's life matters enough to be carried with intention. It is to transform suffering into purpose and chaos into order. Even neuroscience testifies: those who set meaningful goals and labor toward them activate reward circuits more enduring than any fleeting pleasure. The weight of responsibility strengthens rather than crushes; it sculpts character, deepens love, and steadies the mind. The tragedy of our age is not that responsibility is too heavy, but that cowardice convinces us to leave it untouched.

In abandoning responsibility, modern man believes he has chosen freedom, but in truth he has chosen chains. He becomes enslaved to circumstance, to addiction, to despair. And in the silence of his nights, he suspects what he cannot quite name: that the weight he fled from was the very thing that could have given his life dignity. Thus, cowardice is not merely a personal weakness; it is a cultural epidemic, one that hollows the brain, corrodes the soul, and leaves us unfit for the storms of existence. Unless we recover the courage to carry responsibility once more, the modern mind will continue to collapse under the weight of its own evasion.

If cowardice undermines the human will by fleeing responsibility, the cult of shortcuts corrodes it from another direction: by mocking integrity. Every society develops its own euphemism for this practice. In Brazil, one speaks of the jeitinho brasileiro — the little way, the clever maneuver, the art of circumventing rules. Elsewhere, it is dressed in different names: "cutting corners," "gaming the system," or "finding the loophole." Though the words vary, the essence is the same: to pursue advantage without labor, success without merit, appearance without substance.

The shortcut seems harmless at first. A small lie told to avoid a minor consequence, a favor asked to leap over bureaucracy, a rule bent because "everyone else does it." But repeated often enough, these gestures become a culture, and a culture of shortcuts is indistinguishable from corruption. For when truth is negotiable and rules optional, trust evaporates. The student who cheats on an exam may gain a grade, but he loses the formation of his own mind. The politician who pockets public funds may acquire wealth, but he hollows out the very institutions that grant authority. The lover who deceives may enjoy a fleeting conquest, but he corrodes the intimacy that makes love durable. Shortcuts promise efficiency but deliver erosion.

Psychology reveals the deeper danger. Each dishonest act, no matter how small, reshapes the brain's circuitry. Studies show that repeated lying reduces emotional response in the amygdala, the very region that registers guilt. In other words, the more one cheats, the easier it becomes. The shortcut that once caused unease soon feels natural, and integrity begins to seem naïve. Thus dishonesty is not a static flaw but a progressive disease. What begins as convenience becomes character, and what begins as improvisation becomes identity. The brain learns corruption as readily as it learns virtue.

This phenomenon is vividly portrayed in literature. Dostoevsky, in Crime and Punishment, gave us Raskolnikov, who convinced himself that a murder committed for the sake of a higher good would be excusable. Yet the crime did not free him; it enslaved him. His soul, poisoned by the shortcut of justification, could find no peace. So it is with entire societies. When corruption becomes endemic, when every transaction is lubricated by deceit, the collective spirit collapses into suspicion. One no longer expects honesty from a neighbor or leader. Cynicism reigns, and cynicism is but despair clothed in sophistication. The jeitinho may appear playful — a wink, a smile, a clever workaround. But beneath the charm lies a profound contempt for effort. It teaches children that excellence is unnecessary, that perseverance is foolish, that rules are made only to be bent. A young man raised in such an environment may believe he is clever when he deceives, but in truth he is enslaving himself to mediocrity. For genuine achievement requires discipline, and discipline cannot be faked. The shortcut robs him not only of integrity but of the pride that comes only from labor honestly endured.

The consequences extend beyond individual character. In a culture dominated by shortcuts, institutions lose credibility. Meritocracy, already fragile, disintegrates. Why strive if others cheat? Why sacrifice if others are rewarded for deceit? Soon talent flees, ambition dulls, and society stagnates. Innovation requires risk and effort, but a culture addicted to shortcuts avoids both. It prefers the counterfeit over the genuine, the expedient over the enduring. Progress slows, while corruption multiplies. And the citizens, though they may lament the state of affairs, continue to practice the very evasions that perpetuate it.

The link to mental illness may seem less direct, but it is no less real. For integrity is not only a moral virtue; it is a psychological necessity. To live without honesty is to live divided, torn between the mask one wears and the reality one conceals. This division breeds anxiety, for every deception risks exposure; it breeds depression, for a life without authenticity cannot nourish the soul; it breeds addiction, for dishonesty requires constant escape from the conscience it wounds. Thus corruption does not merely damage society; it sickens the individual mind.

Even love, that most intimate of human experiences, cannot survive in an atmosphere of shortcuts. Fidelity demands endurance, communication requires truth, intimacy requires courage. The one who seeks the jeitinho in relationships — hiding betrayal, offering half-truths, feigning commitment — may gain pleasure in the moment, but he loses the trust upon which love is built. In the long run, he is left with fragments: encounters without depth, desires without permanence, connections without meaning. And these fragments, though numerous, cannot satisfy the hunger for belonging that defines our species. Thus, shortcuts in love do not liberate but condemn us to loneliness.

Consider, too, the erosion of self-esteem that follows from living by shortcuts. Pride is not born of ease; it is born of struggle endured. The student who passes an exam through cheating may smile outwardly, but inwardly he knows he has accomplished nothing. The worker who secures a position through connections rather than competence may enjoy the salary, but he cannot enjoy the dignity of merit. Self-esteem requires authenticity, and authenticity cannot be forged by deceit. In this way, shortcuts undermine the very confidence they are meant to preserve.

What, then, is the alternative? It is not the rigid legalism that suffocates life, but the recognition that discipline and honesty are the only soil in which genuine growth occurs. To refuse shortcuts is to accept difficulty, to embrace delay, to endure frustration. But it is also to gain resilience, pride, and authenticity. Neuroscience confirms what philosophy has long taught: sustained effort, rather than easy gain, activates the brain's deepest reward systems. Integrity, though arduous, satisfies more deeply than deceit ever could.

The temptation of shortcuts will never vanish. They appeal to something ancient in the human heart: the desire for reward without suffering, for Eden without toil. Yet every myth reminds us that such desires come at a cost. Prometheus stole fire and was chained; Faust bargained for power and was damned. The modern shortcut may not be so dramatic, but its logic is the same. It offers gain without sacrifice, but the price is hidden: the corruption of character, the collapse of trust, the sickness of the soul.

Thus, the jeitinho is not merely a local habit but a universal danger. It whispers to every society: "Why struggle when you can evade? Why labor when you can feign?" To resist that whisper is difficult, but to surrender is fatal. For when corruption becomes the air we breathe, meaning collapses, responsibility becomes unbearable, and love itself disintegrates. The shortcut, in promising liberation, delivers only decay. And the modern brain, already fragile from cowardice and meaninglessness, finds itself further weakened, unable to anchor itself in truth.

The sickness of our age is not only that we suffer, but that we suffer dishonorably, seeking relief through evasion rather than through endurance. In this, shortcuts and cowardice are twins: both avoid difficulty, both betray responsibility, both leave the soul hollow. And as we will see, such hollowing does not remain moral or cultural alone; it inscribes itself into our neurons, our emotions, our very capacity for love. The shortcut is not only a civic disease; it is a psychological one. Unless resisted, it drags us further into the crisis of the modern mind, where anxiety, depression, and addiction become not aberrations but inevitabilities.

If shortcuts erode integrity and cowardice hollows out courage, then addiction completes the assault by chaining the will itself. It is not new that human beings seek intoxication; wine, opium, and countless other substances have long offered relief from pain or an escape into ecstasy. But what distinguishes our era is not merely the existence of intoxicants — it is their omnipresence, their refinement, and their union with technologies designed to exploit the same vulnerabilities in the human brain. We live in an age where both chemicals and screens, substances and signals, conspire to make addiction not the exception but the expected condition of modern life.

The line between relief and dependence is perilously thin. A drink at night may soothe the nerves, but repeated nightly it becomes ritual, then necessity, and finally enslavement. The cigarette that once calmed anxiety becomes the anxiety that demands another cigarette. The pill prescribed to restore sleep erodes the brain's ability to sleep unaided. Addiction begins as a guest we invite and ends as a master we serve. Neuroscience maps this progression with precision: repeated exposure to intoxicants overstimulates dopamine release, leading to downregulation of receptors. The brain, flooded too often, learns to expect the flood, and in its absence it feels not normality but withdrawal. What began as pleasure becomes torment.

Yet the modern epidemic extends far beyond bottles and powders. Addiction today wears a digital mask. The screen that glows in our palm, the feed that never ends, the game that never concludes — these are not neutral inventions. They are carefully engineered to hijack the same reward systems as cocaine or nicotine. Each notification is a hit of dopamine, each scroll a gamble for novelty, each "like" a micro-dose of social approval. The brain, ancient in its wiring, cannot distinguish between substance and signal; it craves both with equal ferocity. Thus we find ourselves addicted not only to chemicals but to pixels, not only to substances but to symbols.

The consequences seep into every domain of life. Sleep, the first and most essential healer of the brain, collapses under the glow of midnight screens. Intimacy falters when lovers turn toward their devices rather than each other. Attention fragments into shards, unable to sustain the silence in which thought matures. Even ambition withers, for why labor toward distant goals when the screen offers instant gratification? Addiction, whether chemical or digital, is not merely a personal weakness; it is a structural assault upon the conditions necessary for a healthy mind.

Consider the student who cannot study without pausing every few minutes to check a phone, whose evenings stretch into early mornings under the narcotic of streaming platforms. He tells himself he is relaxing, but in truth he is eroding his capacity for sustained attention, the very foundation of learning. Or the professional who unwinds each night with alcohol, at first to ease stress, then to quiet loneliness, and finally to silence despair. He believes he is in control, yet gradually control slips away, until his days are measured not by achievement but by the intervals between doses. Both are captives, though their chains are different.

Addiction, in all its forms, strikes at the root of freedom. For freedom is not the ability to do as one pleases, but the ability to govern one's desires. The addict confuses indulgence with liberty, yet becomes less free with each indulgence. His will shrinks, his courage wanes, his identity dissolves into compulsion. The tragedy is compounded by shame, for the addict knows his chains yet feels powerless to break them. Thus addiction breeds despair, and despair drives deeper addiction — a vicious circle from which many do not emerge.

The link between addiction and mental illness is not incidental but essential. Anxiety grows when the brain, dependent on constant stimulation, can no longer endure stillness. Depression deepens when natural sources of pleasure are overshadowed by the artificial highs of intoxication. Suicide lurks when the pain of withdrawal seems unbearable and the future offers no relief. Addiction is not simply a symptom of despair; it is also its multiplier, amplifying the very illnesses it promises to soothe.

Nor is love spared. Intimacy demands presence, patience, and vulnerability. Yet addiction offers only absence. A partner lost to substances cannot give himself wholly; a partner lost to screens is present in body but absent in soul. Relationships collapse not always from malice but from neglect, from the quiet erosion of attention. Sexuality, too, is distorted by addiction. Pornography, consumed endlessly, conditions desire into unreality, leaving real encounters diminished, and love reduced to performance. Thus addiction undermines not only health but the very bonds that make life bearable.

The cultural implications are immense. A society of addicts is a society without resilience. Citizens preoccupied with consumption cannot muster the discipline for civic duty; parents distracted by screens cannot transmit values to children; workers numbed by substances cannot innovate or endure. Addiction fragments not only individuals but communities, leaving behind a population connected by networks yet alienated in spirit. What once bound people together — family meals, shared rituals, common silence — has been displaced by parallel isolations, each person absorbed in a private intoxication. And yet, perhaps the deepest tragedy is that addiction thrives precisely where meaning has collapsed and responsibility has been abandoned. For the addict is often one who could not endure the emptiness of his days, the weight of his cowardice, the hollowness of his shortcuts. Addiction is not merely an accident; it is the logical refuge of a life unmoored. It offers what society no longer provides: an immediate, if false, sense of purpose. The cigarette tells the hand what to do, the drink dictates the evening, the screen fills the silence. Better a false order than none at all.

To confront addiction, then, is not simply to restrict substances or regulate screens, though such measures matter. It is to confront the void into which these addictions rush. It is to acknowledge that the modern brain, deprived of meaning, responsibility, and authentic intimacy, will seek solace wherever it can. Neuroscience may explain the mechanisms, but culture explains the prevalence. Addiction is the symptom; despair is the disease. Until the deeper wounds are addressed, the chains will only multiply, gilded in new forms but identical in function.

Addiction reminds us of a harsh truth: the mind cannot remain empty. It will be filled, whether with purpose or with poison. A society that fails to offer its citizens meaning, courage, integrity, and love should not be surprised when they turn instead to substances and screens. For the human soul, like the human brain, abhors a vacuum. And in our age, that vacuum is filled not by silence or prayer, not by dreams or duties, but by the endless flicker of distraction and the false comfort of intoxication. Unless this changes, the sick brain will remain our most faithful mirror.

If addiction enslaves the will through intoxication, the cult of comfort weakens it through softness. Never before in human history has life been so carefully padded against hardship. Our homes are heated and cooled to perfection; our food arrives at the door with scarcely a gesture; our entertainments multiply endlessly, requiring no more effort than the flick of a finger. We have succeeded in removing pain, risk, and inconvenience from daily existence to an extent unimaginable to our ancestors. And yet, what we celebrate as progress may also be a form of anesthesia. For in stripping difficulty from life, we have also stripped away the very conditions that strengthen character.

It is tempting to believe that comfort is the natural goal of civilization, that the purpose of progress is to eliminate all suffering. But a closer look at the human psyche reveals another truth: it is not comfort but challenge that shapes us. Muscles grow only when strained, courage only when tested, wisdom only when tempered by adversity. To live without hardship is not to live more fully but to live half-formed, deprived of the trials that mature us. By pursuing comfort at all costs, modern man has achieved ease but forfeited resilience.

The brain itself requires difficulty. Stress, in measured doses, activates pathways that prepare us for future challenges. Psychologists call this "stress inoculation": the process by which small trials build capacity for larger ones. Children who are shielded from all struggle grow fragile, unable to withstand the smallest frustration. Adults who avoid discomfort at every turn lose the ability to endure inevitable setbacks. Neuroscience confirms what every stoic philosopher knew: without friction, the mind dulls. It is through resistance, not ease, that the brain develops resilience.

But the culture of our time insists otherwise. We are told to seek happiness as if it were a permanent state, to demand safety as if it were a right, to avoid difficulty as if it were a pathology. Workplaces promise endless accommodations, schools attempt to eliminate every possibility of failure, and families mistake protection for love. The result is a generation exquisitely sensitive to pain yet poorly equipped to endure it — a population fragile not because it is weak by nature, but because it has been overprotected. What we call compassion may in fact be the breeding ground of despair.

Consider the difference between the soldier who endures the brutal rigor of training and the student who collapses under the weight of a single disappointing grade. The former, though battered, emerges stronger, confident that he can withstand future trials. The latter, though comforted, emerges brittle, convinced that life is unjust at the slightest resistance. This is not a matter of individual weakness but of cultural conditioning. We have mistaken ease for kindness and forgotten that growth demands difficulty. In so doing, we have cultivated fragility on a mass scale.

The implications extend far beyond personal resilience. Comfort erodes ambition. Why labor toward a distant goal when immediate pleasures abound? Why risk failure when safety is assured? The entrepreneur who once dared to sail into uncharted seas now scrolls through digital diversions; the artist who once endured poverty for the sake of vision now seeks viral recognition instead of lasting creation. In a culture dominated by comfort, greatness becomes improbable. We inherit security, but we lose the fire that once built cathedrals, discovered continents, and carved philosophies out of suffering.

Love, too, suffers in a climate of fragility. For intimacy is not maintained by comfort but by the willingness to endure difficulty together. The couple who expects perpetual ease abandons each other at the first quarrel. The partner who cannot tolerate discomfort flees when sacrifice is demanded. Sexuality, reduced to convenience, becomes fragile, incapable of sustaining passion across the seasons of life. Love requires resilience, yet resilience cannot flourish where fragility is the rule. Thus the culture of comfort undermines not only ambition but also intimacy, leaving relationships as brittle as the individuals who form them.

The pursuit of comfort also distorts our relationship with suffering itself. Once regarded as an inevitable part of existence, suffering is now treated as a scandal, an error that must be eliminated at any cost. We medicalize every discomfort, anesthetize every pain, distract ourselves from every silence. But suffering, though painful, is also instructive. It teaches humility, endurance, and compassion. To refuse suffering altogether is to refuse its lessons, leaving us not only unprepared for hardship but also incapable of empathy. A man who has never suffered cannot truly console; a society that refuses to suffer cannot truly grow.

The result of this cultural anesthesia is paradoxical: in trying to eliminate suffering, we have made ourselves more vulnerable to it. Anxiety flourishes in those who cannot tolerate discomfort; depression deepens in those who see every difficulty as a failure; addiction multiplies in those who seek relief from the slightest unease. Suicide, the most tragic of escapes, often appears in precisely those contexts where life is easiest, where suffering is no longer interpreted as meaningful but as intolerable. Thus, the culture of comfort does not prevent despair; it prepares the ground for its expansion.

History offers a stark contrast. Earlier generations endured wars, famines, migrations, and plagues with fewer psychological breakdowns than we witness today in times of peace and abundance. This is not because they were nobler by nature, but because hardship was woven into the fabric of life. Children saw death and learned to accept it; families endured scarcity and learned to share; societies faced crises and learned resilience. Today, by contrast, many reach adulthood without ever confronting true difficulty. When hardship finally arrives — as it always does — they collapse, bewildered that life could betray the promise of perpetual ease.

To resist the cult of comfort is not to glorify suffering but to recognize its necessity. Just as exercise strengthens muscle by stressing it, so too does challenge strengthen the soul. A society that shelters its citizens from every difficulty robs them of resilience. And without resilience, the mind becomes fragile, the mood unstable, the will incapable of enduring. The irony is cruel: by protecting ourselves from pain, we have made ourselves incapable of bearing it.

What, then, is the path forward? It is not to reject progress or embrace needless hardship, but to restore balance. To reintroduce challenge where it has been eliminated, to value endurance as highly as comfort, to teach children not only to avoid pain but to endure it with dignity. We must remember that strength is not inherited but forged, that happiness is not found in perpetual ease but in the confidence that one can withstand adversity. Only then can comfort take its proper place: not as an idol to be worshiped, but as a brief rest earned after labor, a reprieve that strengthens rather than weakens.

The worship of comfort is perhaps the most seductive of our modern idols, for it disguises itself as compassion, progress, even love. But beneath its softness lies fragility, and fragility is the enemy of freedom. For only those who can endure difficulty are truly free; the rest are prisoners of their fear. In the end, the cult of comfort does not spare us suffering — it ensures that when suffering arrives, we will be unprepared. And in that unpreparedness, the sick brain finds its most fertile soil.

If comfort lulls us into fragility, then the death of dreaming seals our fate. For man is not sustained by bread alone, nor even by safety, but by vision. To dream is to imagine a future larger than the present, to stretch the self toward horizons not yet reached, to believe that one's existence may participate in something greater than survival. Without dreams, life collapses into repetition; days blur, years vanish, and existence becomes nothing more than endurance. A society that ceases to dream does not stagnate gently; it decays.

There was a time when dreaming was the natural air of human life. The explorers who set sail for unknown continents, the scientists who peered through crude instruments to discover new worlds, the poets who sought to capture eternity in fragile words — all lived by dreams that reached beyond their circumstances. Their courage was not born of comfort but of vision, a conviction that life could be remade, enlarged, redeemed by striving. Suffering was endured because it was believed to serve something higher. Hardship was accepted because it was the price of greatness.

Today, such vision has grown rare. We are told instead to dream modestly, to set goals within the narrow confines of career, consumption, and social visibility. Ambition is reduced to accumulation: the next promotion, the larger home, the enviable vacation. Imagination is replaced by simulation: rather than create, we consume images of others' creations, scrolling endlessly through digital galleries of borrowed lives. Even rebellion has been commodified, packaged into trends that expire as quickly as they appear. The dreamer, once admired as a visionary, is now often dismissed as naïve, impractical, even delusional.

The psychological cost is immense. Neuroscience teaches that the brain's default mode network, active during daydreaming and imagination, is essential for envisioning the future and planning meaningful goals. When this capacity is underused — when individuals cease to imagine futures beyond the immediate — the result is not neutrality but despair. Without dreams, the present becomes unbearable, for it offers no path forward. Depression feeds upon this void, whispering that tomorrow will be no different from today, that no effort can alter the trajectory of life. To cease dreaming is to invite despair to become permanent.

Consider the young adult who, after years of study, enters the workforce only to discover that his ambitions have been narrowed to mere survival. He no longer dreams of transforming the world or even his own community; he dreams only of making rent, of distracting himself on weekends, of enduring until retirement. Each day repeats the last, and he grows restless without knowing why. Or the woman who, surrounded by conveniences and comforts, nonetheless feels a gnawing emptiness. She scrolls through images of others' lives, mistaking envy for aspiration, yet she cannot name a vision for her own. Both suffer not from lack of opportunity but from lack of dreaming.

The absence of dreams corrodes not only ambition but love. For love, too, requires imagination. To commit oneself to another is to dream together of a shared future, to believe that two lives intertwined can create something neither could alone. When imagination withers, relationships falter. Partners see only the present irritations, the daily inconveniences, the fragility of desire. Without the dream of a future (a home, a family, a life of meaning together) intimacy collapses into transaction, passion into boredom. The death of dreaming robs love of its most essential element: the vision of tomorrow.

It is no accident that in societies where dreaming has withered, fertility declines, marriages dissolve, and loneliness spreads. A population that cannot imagine a future larger than the present will not invest in families, in communities, in posterity. It will seek only short-term pleasure, immediate security, fleeting distraction. The result is a society of individuals connected by networks but disconnected in purpose, living side by side yet dreaming no common dream. Civilization itself requires vision, and without it, decline is inevitable.

Dreaming, however, is not mere fantasy. It demands courage and action. The dreamer who refuses to act becomes a prisoner of illusion, but the dreamer who acts transforms both himself and his world. What we see today is not only the death of dreaming but the death of doing. Too many are content to imagine vaguely without pursuing concretely, to talk of change without laboring for it, to live as spectators of life rather than its participants. This passivity, disguised as contentment, breeds despair. For the soul knows when it has betrayed its own visions, and that betrayal festers in silence.

Here again addiction conspires with despair. For substances and screens offer the counterfeit of dreaming: stimulation without vision, novelty without direction, excitement without progress. The brain, deprived of genuine imagination, settles for artificial highs. But the satisfaction fades quickly, leaving behind only emptiness and dependence. Addiction and the death of dreaming are thus twin afflictions: one replaces vision with intoxication, the other with distraction. Both end in despair, for both deny the soul the horizon it requires.

The loss of dreaming also erodes self-esteem. To respect oneself is to know that one's life is moving toward something meaningful, that one's sacrifices serve a greater end. Without this conviction, pride vanishes. A man may achieve wealth, recognition, or even comfort, but if he has ceased to dream, he will sense the futility of his gains. His achievements will taste of ash, for they serve no vision beyond themselves. Thus, despair does not come from failure alone but also from success without purpose.

What, then, is required to revive dreaming? Not the naive fantasies of instant gratification, but the patient courage to imagine futures worth suffering for. Dreams must be large enough to justify sacrifice, enduring enough to outlast disappointment, and rooted enough to inspire action. They need not be grandiose; even the dream of raising a child with love, of cultivating a craft with excellence, of building a community with fidelity can sustain a soul against despair. What matters is not the scale but the authenticity of the vision. For in dreaming authentically, man affirms that his life is more than endurance; it is creation.

The death of dreaming is perhaps the quietest of modern tragedies, for it rarely announces itself with drama. It appears instead in monotony, in passivity, in the subtle conviction that nothing new is possible. But beneath its silence lies devastation. Without dreams, anxiety has no antidote, depression has no rival, and addiction has no competitor. To cease dreaming is to cease becoming. And when becoming halts, life itself begins to rot.

If meaning has collapsed, responsibility has been abandoned, shortcuts have corrupted integrity, addictions have enslaved the will, comfort has bred fragility, and dreaming has withered, then nowhere do these afflictions converge more visibly than in love. For love is not merely an ornament to life; it is the crucible in which the deepest truths of human existence are tested. It demands responsibility, courage, honesty, and vision — the very virtues our culture neglects. And when these virtues are absent, intimacy falters, desire fragments, and the sacred bond between two persons dissolves into convenience. Peterson has often argued that responsibility is the bedrock of meaning, and nowhere is this clearer than in relationships. To love another is not simply to feel desire or affection; it is to take upon oneself the responsibility for their well-being, to promise stability even when the storms of life rage. Yet in an age dominated by cowardice, many recoil from such responsibility. They wish for the pleasures of intimacy without its burdens, for the warmth of companionship without the demands of sacrifice. The result is fragile unions, partnerships abandoned at the first sign of difficulty, and a generation increasingly distrustful of permanence. Love without responsibility becomes lust, and lust, though intoxicating, cannot sustain the soul.

Honesty, too, is essential. Peterson warns that lies, even small ones, corrode the soul and relationships alike, for they replace reality with a counterfeit. Love can survive quarrels, disappointment, even betrayal — but it cannot survive deception. Yet in a culture steeped in shortcuts and appearances, dishonesty becomes habitual. We present curated versions of ourselves on screens, edit our words to preserve comfort, evade painful truths in order to maintain peace. But peace purchased by deceit is fragile; it fractures the moment reality intrudes. Intimacy requires truth, and truth requires courage. Without it, relationships are built on sand.

The imbalance between order and chaos, which Peterson sees as the fundamental tension of life, also appears in love. A relationship demands both: order in the form of stability, commitment, and trust; chaos in the form of passion, spontaneity, and growth. Too much order and love becomes rigid, lifeless routine; too much chaos and it dissolves into instability. Yet modern culture, obsessed with novelty and afraid of permanence, leans heavily toward chaos. The perpetual search for new experiences, new partners, new thrills undermines the discipline of building a shared order. Couples lose the patience to cultivate stability, forgetting that it is precisely within the structure of long-term commitment that the richest depths of intimacy unfold. Addiction compounds these difficulties. Digital distractions, pornography, and substances erode the capacity for presence. The partner absorbed by a glowing screen may be physically near yet emotionally absent; the one enslaved to substances may oscillate between craving and withdrawal, unable to offer steadiness. Pornography, in particular, distorts sexuality by conditioning desire toward fantasy rather than reality, making real encounters feel inadequate. Peterson has spoken of how the corruption of sexual relationships weakens not only individuals but society itself, for families — the basic unit of civilization — are founded upon intimate trust. When that trust falters, the entire social fabric trembles.

Comfort and fragility also warp intimacy. A relationship, like any meaningful endeavor, requires endurance through difficulty. There will be quarrels, disappointments, illnesses, failures. But a culture that worships ease and safety breeds partners unwilling to withstand such trials. At the first sign of conflict, they withdraw; at the first demand of sacrifice, they depart. They seek comfort rather than growth, forgetting that true love is forged precisely in the fires of difficulty. Without resilience, intimacy becomes shallow, unable to withstand the ordinary tempests of life.

The death of dreaming also strikes at love's core. To love another is to imagine a future together — a home, a family, a shared life that transcends the present. But when individuals cease to dream, relationships are stripped of vision. Partners see only the present irritations, the mundane routines, the fragility of desire. Without the horizon of a shared future, intimacy collapses into transaction: companionship for convenience, sexuality for gratification, affection for utility. Such unions cannot sustain the human longing for permanence, for transcendence. They may last for months or years, but they do not endure in the way the soul craves.

The consequences are evident in demographic decline across much of the developed world: fertility rates plummet, marriages dissolve, loneliness proliferates. These are not merely economic trends but spiritual symptoms. A society that cannot foster enduring love and family is a society that has lost its foundation. Peterson emphasizes that family, though demanding, is one of the deepest sources of meaning. Children, he insists, anchor adults in responsibility, sacrifice, and hope for the future. But when love disintegrates, families fracture, and the next generation inherits not stability but confusion. The sickness of intimacy becomes the sickness of civilization.

This collapse reverberates through self-esteem as well. For to be loved truly — not for appearances, not for convenience, but for one's whole being — is to receive the deepest affirmation possible. Without such love, individuals seek validation elsewhere: in status, in possessions, in the fickle approval of strangers. Social media, with its endless stream of "likes" and fleeting attention, becomes a counterfeit intimacy, momentarily soothing but ultimately hollow. The result is a generation anxious about their worth, depressed by their solitude, addicted to distractions that cannot satisfy. Love, once the fortress against despair, has itself become fragile.

And yet, the paradox remains: we long for intimacy even as we sabotage it. The very culture that undermines love is also obsessed with it, producing endless songs, films, and stories about connection. This longing testifies that intimacy is not a luxury but a necessity of human life. To be deprived of love is to be deprived of oxygen. But to sustain love requires the virtues we have neglected: responsibility, honesty, endurance, vision. Without them, our longing collapses into disappointment, and disappointment into despair.

The disintegration of love and intimacy is not a peripheral issue; it is the culmination of all the modern maladies we have traced. Meaninglessness, cowardice, corruption, addiction, comfort, fragility, and the death of dreaming — each strikes at love's foundations, and together they topple it. The result is a society where relationships dissolve, families fracture, and loneliness becomes endemic. And in this loneliness, the sick brain flourishes: anxiety sharpens, depression deepens, suicidality spreads. For when even love cannot sustain us, what remains to hold us against the weight of existence?

Love demands more of us than comfort or convenience, more than cowardice or shortcuts, more than addiction or distraction. It demands the courage to face responsibility, the honesty to speak truth, the endurance to withstand hardship, the vision to dream together of a future. In neglecting these, we have not only weakened our relationships but sickened our very minds. To heal the sick brain, we must begin here: by restoring love not as a fleeting pleasure but as the highest responsibility, the most courageous act, the most enduring source of meaning. Without such restoration, the crisis of the modern mind will not abate.

We have walked through the main troubles of our time, and though they appear in different shapes, they all circle back to the same point: we have forgotten what it means to live with weight. Life without meaning, without responsibility, without honesty, without resilience, without dreams, without love — it leaves the brain fragile and the heart restless. And when the brain is fragile and the heart restless, anxiety, depression, addiction, and even suicide stop being rare tragedies and start becoming ordinary outcomes.

Think of it like this: if you plant a tree in weak soil, no amount of sunlight will make it grow strong. Our society has become that weak soil. Comfort without courage, shortcuts without truth, distractions without silence — these are the conditions in which roots fail to take hold. And so, when storms come, the tree falls. The storms themselves are not new; hardship, grief, and suffering have always been part of life. What has changed is that our soil has thinned.

And perhaps the saddest thing is how these problems wound the places that once gave life its deepest sweetness: our love, our friendships, our families. When distraction replaces presence, when cowardice replaces commitment, when comfort replaces endurance, intimacy loses its strength. We want to love, we want to be loved, but we forget that love is less about feeling good in the moment and more about standing tall together when life gets hard.

Jordan Peterson often says that meaning is found not in chasing happiness but in carrying responsibility. That line might sound heavy at first, but it's also liberating. Because the moment you take responsibility — for your health, your work, your family, your love — you stop floating and start standing. You discover that suffering can be endured if it leads somewhere, that dreams can be pursued if you are willing to sacrifice, and that love can last if you are willing to fight for it. None of this is easy, but perhaps easy was never the point.

What we see now is a mirror. Anxiety, depression, and addiction are not just private illnesses; they are reflections of how we have been living collectively. They show us the cost of forgetting meaning, courage, truth, resilience, dreams, and love. And if the mirror is painful, that is not a reason to look away. It is a reason to finally ask the harder questions: what makes a brain sick? What happens, biologically and psychologically, when these conditions press down on us? And more importantly, how do we find the way back?

That is where we must go next. We have traced the social currents; now we will descend into the brain itself, to see how these forces take shape in neurons, synapses, and circuits. For the crisis of the modern mind is not only cultural but biological, not only philosophical but medical. And to heal it, we must learn how the brain becomes sick — and how it can be restored.

This is the crisis of the modern mind: a ceaseless motion that mistakes accumulation for meaning, and a restless anxiety that confuses noise for vitality. But the consequences of such a life are not borne in the abstract alone. They carve themselves into the very fabric of the brain. Every hurried indulgence, every unexamined desire, every abandonment of purpose leaves its trace upon the nervous system, as if culture itself were etching its disquiet into biology. What once seemed merely a moral disorientation now reveals itself as a physiological wound: the sick brain, formed at the crossroads where society's illusions meet the vulnerabilities of human nature. To understand this affliction, we must descend further — from the surface of cultural despair into the hidden mechanisms of the mind, where chemistry and memory conspire to shape disorder.

CHAPTER 3

What Makes a Brain Sick?

The Fragile Balance of the Brain

The human brain survives and thrives by maintaining a fragile balance. Our minds are constantly performing a high-wire act between opposite poles – excitation and inhibition, arousal and rest, stress and recovery. In a healthy state, these forces exist in equilibrium, like a well-balanced seesaw. The main excitatory neurotransmitter glutamate pushes neural activity forward (the "gas pedal"), while GABA (gamma-aminobutyric acid) applies the "brakes" as the primary inhibitory transmitter. Indeed, doctors describe glutamate and GABA as an "on" and "off" switch of the brain – and a delicate balance between them is required for normal function. Too much excitation without enough inhibition can lead to seizures, anxiety, or manic energy; too much inhibition leads to sedation, depression, or cognitive slowing. The brain's well-being depends on this dynamic equilibrium, ensuring that every surge has a counter-buffer and every signal has a modulator.

This principle of balance extends beyond neurotransmitters. Our entire nervous system oscillates between states of heightened arousal and restorative calm. The sympathetic "fight-or-flight" response that floods us with adrenaline and cortisol is meant to be balanced by the parasympathetic "rest-and-digest" response that calms us down. Similarly, periods of intense focus or wakefulness must be followed by sleep and mental downtime. In essence, stability emerges from the interplay of opposites. As one insightful reflection put it, "extremes are two sides of the same coin" – like day and night, each state gives meaning to its counterpart. If we never experienced fatigue, we couldn't value rest; without stress, relief would be meaningless. The brain, in its wisdom, constantly toggles between these poles, striving to maintain stability through change – a process scientists term allostasis. Allostasis is the brain's way of achieving equilibrium not by staying static, but by actively adjusting to whatever life throws at it. For example, your brain will raise your heart rate and blood pressure in the morning to energize you, then lower them at night so you can sleep – changing set-points to keep internal conditions stable. It's like a smart thermostat that anticipates the temperature and constantly recalibrates to keep the house comfortable.

However, this balancing act is precarious. Under conditions of chronic stress or overstimulation, the normal allostatic adjustments can overshoot, leading to wear and tear on the system. Think of a machine forced to run at full throttle with no cool-down period – components will start to break. In the brain, chronic stress creates an allostatic load – essentially the cumulative "wear and tear" from repeated stress adjustments. Over time, this load can tip the balance toward disease. The stress hormones that are protective in the short run (cortisol, adrenaline) become harmful when constantly elevated. They trigger chemical imbalances, disturb our circadian rhythms, and can even atrophy brain structures like the memory centers. In the words of neuroscientist Bruce McEwen, chronic stress literally reshapes the brain: in anxiety, depression, or PTSD, "allostatic load takes the form of chemical imbalances as well as perturbations in the diurnal rhythm, and, in some cases, atrophy of brain structures." For instance, those suffering from long-term trauma or hardship often have a shrunken hippocampus (a brain region vital for memory) due to sustained cortisol exposure killing neurons or stunting new growth. The brain's attempt to adapt through change backfires – the allostatic process becomes inefficient and damaging, a state termed allostatic overload. Metaphorically, the brain's delicate seesaw is smashed to the ground on one side.

Crucially, many mental illnesses can be seen as manifestations of this broken balance. Prolonged stress or overstimulation can push neural circuits out of their optimal ranges. Without enough time in "rest and recover" mode, the brain's excitatory signals run rampant, depleting neurotransmitters and exhausting neural pathways. It's no coincidence that people under unrelenting stress often report feeling "wired and tired" – simultaneously agitated and depleted. If the system remains out of balance for too long, it predisposes to illness. For example, chronic stress and sleep deprivation might precipitate an anxiety disorder in one person or major depression in another. The exact outcome varies, but the common thread is that the brain's fragile equilibrium has been destabilized. At the extreme, a person might experience a nervous breakdown – essentially the brain hitting an emergency reset after being pushed past its adaptive limits. Trauma is another profound disruptor: a single catastrophic event (or cumulative micro-traumas) can permanently alter the balance between fear circuits and calming circuits, leaving the person in a constant state of "high alert" even in safe environments. The balance between 'on' and 'off' has been reset to a new, unhealthy point. Modern neuroscience has shown that such imbalance isn't just metaphorical – it's visible in the brain. Functional brain scans of PTSD patients, for instance, show overactive amygdalae (the brain's threat detectors) flaring even at mild stimuli, as if the brain's fear switch is stuck in the "on" position. In depression, by contrast, brain networks for reward and motivation can become under-active – the neural "volume knob" for pleasure is turned down too low, resulting in emotional numbness and anhedonia.

In short, the healthy mind lives by a golden mean: oscillating between extremes but avoiding either extreme for too long. Stability through rhythmic change. When that rhythm is lost – when the fragile balance of the brain is disrupted by chronic stress, trauma, or biological factors – mental illness can emerge. But to truly understand these illnesses, we must peek under the hood at the brain's key systems and see how they function in health and go awry in sickness.

Key Brain Systems Involved in Mood and Mental Health

The brain is the most complex orchestra on Earth, and our mood and behavior emerge from the harmonies (and discords) of many neural instruments. Four major "circuits" are especially relevant to mental health: the limbic system, the prefrontal cortex, the brain's reward pathways, and the HPA axis (stress response system). Each plays a distinct role in regulating emotions, motivation, and reactions to stress. When these systems run smoothly, we experience fear when appropriate, soothe ourselves after, pursue rewards in moderation, and cope with stress adaptively. But when they malfunction or fall out of balance, the result can be anxiety, depression, impulsivity, or addiction. Let's briefly tour these systems, using some metaphors to illustrate their roles, and see what happens when things go wrong.

The Limbic System: Fear and Memory in the Inner Sanctuary

Deep in the brain lies the limbic system, an evolutionarily ancient region responsible for emotion, motivation, and memory. Key players here are the amygdala and the hippocampus – often called the brain's "fear center" and "memory center," respectively. The amygdala is an almond-shaped cluster of neurons that acts like a smoke alarm for threats. If you see a snake or hear a sudden bang, it's your amygdala that ignites the flash of fear before you even consciously register the danger. It triggers the fight-or-flight response – sweating, heart racing, focus sharpened. This little structure is exquisitely tuned to anything that might harm you, and it works with lightning speed to keep you safe. The hippocampus, curled beside the amygdala, is like the brain's archivist or librarian – it helps form new memories and contextualizes fear by providing background information. If the amygdala is the alarm, the hippocampus writes down what happened and notes the where and when. It's critical for learning from experience (so you remember where the snake was and avoid it next time) and for distinguishing past from present (reminding you that a current loud bang is just New Year's fireworks, not a gunshot from that war you survived).

In a healthy state, the amygdala and hippocampus work in tandem with higher brain areas to manage fear appropriately. You feel fear when needed, but you also extinguish fear when safety returns (with the hippocampus signaling "all clear, that was then, this is now"). Memory of danger is stored without overwhelming you. However, in anxiety disorders and PTSD this circuit goes awry. The amygdala can become overactive and hypersensitive, like a smoke alarm that goes off at the slightest toast burning. Studies have found that patients with PTSD show greater amygdala activation than controls in response to even subtle reminders of trauma – e.g. a faint sound or a single word can trigger a full fear response. Their threat-detector is essentially jammed in the "on" position, flooding them with terror at benign cues. Meanwhile, the hippocampus often shrinks under chronic stress and trauma. Elevated cortisol over time is toxic to hippocampal neurons and can inhibit new neuron formation. Brain scans of trauma survivors and people with major depression have repeatedly shown a smaller hippocampus – on the order of 10–15% reduced volume in depression, for example. This atrophy is thought to contribute to memory problems (difficulty forming new memories or recalling positive memories) and to an impaired ability to contextualize fear. In PTSD, a weakened hippocampus may fail to remind the person that "that was then, you are safe now," so the past invades the present in the form of flashbacks and constant dread. The limbic system, instead of serving us by producing appropriate fear and encoding memories, becomes a source of pathology: persistent anxiety, intrusive memories, and emotional overwhelm. An overactive amygdala can produce free-floating anxiety and panic attacks (imagine feeling afraid without knowing why – the alarm with no clear fire). And a weakened hippocampus leaves one at the mercy of those alarms, unable to properly file away traumatic events as memories in the past. This is why healing from trauma often involves calming the amygdala and strengthening the hippocampus (for instance, through certain therapies or even medications that promote new brain cell growth). It's a delicate balance: too much fear versus too little, too vivid a memory versus too blank. The limbic system's equilibrium is central to our emotional stability.

The Prefrontal Cortex: Planning, Control, and the Voice of Reason

If the limbic system is the emotional engine, the prefrontal cortex (PFC) is the steering wheel. Located right behind your forehead, the PFC is the most evolved part of the brain – often described as the CEO, conductor, or executive that manages the rest of the brain. This region enables our uniquely human abilities: long-term planning, logical reasoning, impulse control, concentration, and decision-making based on goals rather than immediate impulses. It's the mental brake pedal that can override the amygdala's knee-jerk fear or the urge to eat a second piece of cake. A well-functioning prefrontal cortex allows us to pause and think: to consider consequences, to act in line with our values, and to modulate our emotions with rational thought. For example, if you're angry at someone, your PFC helps you not punch them in the face – it weighs the consequences and applies the brakes on your aggressive impulse. It's also the source of willpower that helps you get up for work even when you'd rather sleep, or stick to a difficult task because you know it's important.

In many mental illnesses, this top-down control system is underactive or dysregulated, leading to symptoms of poor judgment, impulsivity, or overwhelming emotions. A classic example comes from the famous case of Phineas Gage, a 19th-century railroad worker who survived an accident that drove an iron rod through his skull, obliterating much of his left prefrontal cortex. Gage lived, but his personality changed radically: the responsible, mild-mannered man became irreverent, impulsive, and unable to stick to plans. As one early account described, he became "fitful, irreverent, indulging at times in the grossest profanity... impatient of restraint or advice when it conflicts with his desires." Neurologists often summarize his condition by saying Gage lost his inhibition and self-control – in modern terms, damage to his PFC left him "disinhibited", unable to restrain impulses or adhere to social norms. This striking case was one of the first clues that the prefrontal cortex is vital for impulse control, decision-making, and moderating social behavior. In essence, Phineas Gage demonstrated what happens when the brain's "conductor" goes offline: the symphony of the brain turns chaotic.

(Notably, Gage did partially recover over time – a testament to the brain's plasticity and ability to rewire, which we'll discuss later.)

In less extreme ways, prefrontal dysfunction is seen in disorders like ADHD (poor attention and impulse control), bipolar disorder during manic episodes (reckless behavior and reduced judgment), and even in depression. In fact, depression has been consistently associated with impaired prefrontal cortex activity. Scans of people with major depression show that parts of the PFC (especially the dorsolateral and dorsomedial regions involved in cognitive control) are often underactive, while emotion-generating regions run amok. This may explain why depressed individuals struggle with concentration, decision-making, and escaping negative thought loops – the brain's "thinking captain" isn't exerting normal control to shift thoughts or initiate hopeful action. They can get stuck in ruminative, automatic patterns. Similarly, in anxiety disorders, the PFC's regulation of the amygdala may be compromised, so rationally knowing "this is not a threat" doesn't fully quiet the fear. On the flip side, some disorders (like obsessive-compulsive disorder) might involve over-activity in certain frontal regions leading to over-control, but generally the theme in many mood and impulse disorders is a loss of prefrontal regulatory strength. We see evidence of this in addiction as well: chronically addicted individuals often have reduced activity in the prefrontal cortex, correlating with their diminished self-control in resisting drug use. In active addiction or during cravings, blood flow to prefrontal areas drops while more primitive reward regions light up, indicating that impulsive desire is overwhelming the rational brakes. Overall, an underpowered prefrontal cortex is like a weak muscle – it tires easily, allowing impulses and emotions to run ahead. Strengthening this "muscle" through practices like mindfulness or cognitive training can improve self-regulation, much as rehabilitation helped Phineas Gage relearn some self-control. The balance between the "go" signals of impulse (generated by deeper brain areas) and the "stop" signals of the PFC is crucial. When the balance tilts too far toward impulsivity, we lose our governing capacity and risk behaviors that harm ourselves or others.

The Reward System: Dopamine, Desire, and Addiction's Hijack

Why do we seek certain experiences and avoid others? Why do some people fall into addiction while others do not? The answers lie in the brain's reward system, a network of regions that uses the neurotransmitter dopamine to reinforce behaviors. This circuit's hub is the mesolimbic pathway, running from the ventral tegmental area (VTA) in the midbrain to the nucleus accumbens (NAc) deep in the forebrain. You can think of this pathway as the brain's motivation highway – whenever you do something that the brain interprets as beneficial or pleasurable (eating tasty food, having social interaction, accomplishing a goal), the VTA releases a burst of dopamine into the nucleus accumbens, creating a sensation of pleasure or satisfaction. This is the brain's way of saying "Yes, that was good, do that again!" Evolution wired this system to reinforce survival-enhancing activities like eating, mating, exploring, and bonding with others. Dopamine, importantly, is not just about pleasure – it's about wanting and motivation. It's the spark that makes you desire to repeat an action. In a normal context, this system ensures we seek food when hungry, strive for achievement, and enjoy life's rewards in a balanced way. However, the reward system is highly vulnerable to hijacking. Certain substances (like drugs of abuse: cocaine, meth, opioids) and even behaviors (gambling, video games, etc.) can trigger unnaturally large surges of dopamine, far beyond what normal life experiences produce. It's as if these artificial rewards smash the "pleasure button" in the brain, flooding the nucleus accumbens with dopamine. The result is an intense high – and a reinforcement signal that is too strong for the brain's balance to handle. In response to these repeated dopamine floods, the brain tries to restore equilibrium by downregulating its dopamine response. Receptors for dopamine in the reward circuit may become less sensitive or decrease in number, attempting to put the brakes on the excessive stimulation. Over time, this adaptation leads to tolerance (needing more of the substance to get the same effect) and a diminished ability to feel pleasure from natural rewards. In other words, as addiction develops, the dopamine balance tilts: the person feels flat, depressed, or unmotivated when not using the drug because their baseline dopamine activity has been suppressed by the brain's adaptations. Normal joys – a sunset, a meal, socializing – don't register much, because the reward system has been numbed. Pleasure becomes narrow and elusive, obtainable reliably only through the addictive substance or behavior, which now isn't even causing euphoria so much as just briefly alleviating the dopamine-deprived misery. This state is often described by addicted individuals as "needing a fix just to feel normal."

Even outside of addiction, dysfunctions of the reward system are implicated in mental health. In major depression, for instance, many patients experience anhedonia – the inability to feel pleasure or motivation. Neuroimaging studies show that depressed individuals often have blunted activation of the nucleus accumbens and related reward circuitry when exposed to positive stimuli, compared to healthy people. Essentially, the brain's reward pathway is under-active – the dopamine release that should occur to signal interest or enjoyment is diminished. One meta-analysis found decreased functional connectivity within the brain's reward network to be a robust feature of depression, suggesting a physical correlation of the patient's subjective "nothing feels rewarding" experience. In line with this, many modern treatments for depression (from certain medications to deep brain stimulation in experimental cases) aim to boost dopamine or re-engage the reward circuit to restore motivation and pleasure. On the other end, bipolar mania can involve an overactive reward system – manic individuals often have excessive goal-directed activity, impulsive pleasure-seeking, and an inflated sense of reward (they might pursue risky investments or activities because their brain is effectively screaming "this will be great!" without caution). So, the balance in dopamine signaling is key: too little and life is gray and unmotivating; too much (or too easily triggered) and one can lose judgment or become addicted to highs. The reward system is like the brain's carrot-on-a-stick – when properly calibrated it keeps us moving forward in life, but if the carrot is too powerful or the stick too weak, we either chase destructive rewards or stop moving altogether.

The HPA Axis: Stress, Cortisol, and the Burnout Response

Last but not least, we come to the HPA axis – the hypothalamic–pituitary–adrenal axis – which is the body's central stress response system. If the amygdala is the smoke alarm, the HPA axis is the sprinkler system that kicks in to address the fire. It is a hormonal feedback loop: when your brain perceives stress or danger, the hypothalamus (H) releases CRH (corticotropin-releasing hormone), which signals the pituitary gland (P) to secrete ACTH (adrenocorticotropic hormone) into the bloodstream, which in turn prompts the adrenal glands (A), perched atop your kidneys, to release cortisol (the primary stress hormone in humans). Cortisol surges through the body to help mobilize energy – raising blood sugar, increasing metabolism, sharpening attention – basically putting you into "fight or flight" mode to cope with the challenge. In the short term, this response is adaptive and critical for survival. Cortisol also feeds back to the brain (binding to glucocorticoid receptors) to help shut down the stress response when the threat passes, maintaining homeostasis via negative feedback. Under healthy circumstances, the HPA axis activation is brief and appropriate: you encounter a stressor, mount a stress response (cortisol spike), then once it's handled, cortisol levels drop and your body returns to baseline.

Trouble arises when the HPA axis is overactive or stuck "on" due to chronic stress. If someone is under persistent psychological stress – say, a child in an abusive household or an adult in a warzone or an extremely pressured job – the HPA axis can become hyper-reactive and dysregulated. It's like a fire alarm that keeps ringing and a sprinkler that never fully shuts off, soaking the system. Chronically elevated cortisol can wreak havoc on both brain and body. It can impair immune function, contribute to weight gain and high blood pressure, and crucially, it affects the brain regions we've discussed: prolonged cortisol exposure can damage the hippocampus (leading to memory problems) and alter amygdala and prefrontal function (skewing emotional regulation). In fact, more than 40–60% of patients with major depression show evidence of HPA axis overactivity, such as elevated cortisol levels or a failure to suppress cortisol after a dexamethasone challenge test. This hypercortisolemia in depression is associated with cognitive impairment and a more severe course of illness. Essentially, many depressed individuals are living in a state of chronic stress response – their bodies act like there's an ongoing emergency that never abates. This can manifest as feelings of constant tension, poor sleep (since cortisol disturbs sleep cycles), anxiety agitation, and even physical symptoms. In anxiety disorders, a similar pattern is often present: the stress response is over-engaged. People with generalized anxiety, for instance, often have elevated cortisol throughout the day, as if their internal alarm never quiets. Over time, this can lead to burnout – the system may get exhausted and cortisol levels can flatten (which is another problem, as seen in some PTSD cases where the system "crashes"). Another aspect is how early life adversity programs the HPA axis. Traumatic experiences in childhood – such as abuse, neglect, or chronic fear – can calibrate a person's stress response to be hyper-sensitive for life. Research shows that childhood trauma significantly increases the risk of adult mental illness, in part by inducing long-term dysfunction in the HPA axis. In one long-running study, adults who had traumatic childhoods showed a more reactive cortisol response to stress and higher incidence of depression and PTSD later on. In essence, their brains learned early that the world is dangerous, and their stress machinery got stuck in high gear. This is a prime example of the brain's plasticity working in a maladaptive way – the developing HPA axis overshoots in adapting to a toxic environment, and that new set-point becomes a liability when the person is in a normal environment. The balance between stress and calm is hard to regain. The HPA axis can also affect other systems: for example, excessive cortisol can deplete certain neurotransmitters and promote inflammation, which has been linked to depression as well. On a positive note, treatments targeting the HPA axis (like certain antidepressants, psychotherapy techniques like trauma-focused CBT, or even emerging drugs that block specific stress receptors) show promise in restoring a healthier balance. The key point is that a properly functioning HPA axis is like a well-tuned thermostat: it turns on the heat when needed and turns it off when things are warm enough. In mental illness, that thermostat often breaks – either blasting stress hormones non-stop (anxiety, melancholic depression) or becoming erratic. The result is a body and brain flooded with stress chemicals or unable to mount a proper stress response when actually needed. Healing often involves resetting this system, through both biological and behavioral interventions (learning stress management, processing trauma, etc.).

Having explored these four systems – the limbic network for fear/emotion, the prefrontal cortex for control, the reward circuitry for motivation, and the HPA axis for stress regulation – a pattern emerges: mental health is a tightrope walk of balance. In each case, illness tends to involve doing too much or too little of something: feeling too much fear or too little pleasure, acting on too many impulses or none at all, having stress hormones too high or (in burnout) too low. Our brains strive for a Goldilocks zone in everything. And this brings us to an even more humbling truth: given the right (or wrong) circumstances, anyone's brain can lose its balance. No one is invulnerable to mental illness, because we all share these same fragile systems.

Vulnerability and Universality: Why No One Is Immune

One of the central messages in modern psychiatry is that mental illness does not reflect a personal weakness or a rare flaw – it reflects the human condition under strain. We all have the same basic brain architecture discussed above, and thus we all have the capacity for these systems to malfunction if pushed beyond their limits. In fact, an expansive global study in 2023 found that one out of every two people will develop a mental health disorder in their lifetime. That is 50% of humanity – literally every other person. This striking statistic underlines the universality of mental illness: if it's not you, it's someone you love. And even those who never cross the diagnostic threshold will still experience periods of significant psychological suffering, whether it's grief, anxiety, trauma, or extreme stress. The potential for things to go wrong lives in all of our brains. Just as everyone's physical body can fall ill or break under certain conditions, everyone's mind has breaking points. The brain's balancing mechanisms are robust, but not unbreakable.

Of course, individuals vary in vulnerability. Some people seem to weather extraordinary stress with minimal fallout, while others develop depression or anxiety under pressures that seem mild. Why is this? Research points to a combination of genetics, early life experiences, and current environment as key factors. On the genetic side, we know that mental illnesses tend to run in families, indicating a heritable component. However, genes usually don't act alone; they interact with life events. A famous example is the serotonin transporter gene (5-HTTLPR). A study by Caspi et al. (2003) showed that people with a certain variant of this gene (the "short" allele) were much more likely to become depressed after stressful life events than those with the long allele. In those with two short alleles, rates of depression spiked as the number of adverse events increased, whereas those with two long alleles were comparatively protected – as if genetics gave them a thicker cushion against stress. Notably, if no stressful events occurred, having the risky gene didn't cause depression on its own. This illustrates the diathesis-stress model: genes may load the gun, but the environment pulls the trigger. Many similar gene-environment interactions have been explored, from genes affecting dopamine or neuroplasticity to genes in the HPA axis. The takeaway is that some of us are born with more sensitive circuitry – perhaps an amygdala that's easily set off, or slower serotonin production, etc. – and thus are at higher risk if we encounter hardships. But often those same genes might confer advantages in a gentler environment (for instance, making someone more empathetic or driven). This is why we say vulnerability is not destiny; it's a factor, not a fate.

Childhood experiences are incredibly important in shaping vulnerability. As discussed, early trauma can supercharge the stress response and embed maladaptive patterns that echo throughout life. The developing brain is impressionable ("plastic"), so a child who endures abuse, neglect, or serious loss may have an emotional foundation of fear or low self-worth that predisposes them to later breakdowns. The landmark Adverse Childhood Experiences (ACE) studies found a dose-response relationship – the more types of adversity (e.g. violence, poverty, parental substance abuse) someone suffered as a child, the higher their risk for everything from depression and suicide to heart disease in adulthood. Long periods of instability in our formative years – times when our psyche is not in sync with what society expects or needs – can literally cause hormonal and neuronal imbalances that persist. For example, a teenager who faces constant bullying and isolation (being "out of sync" with peers) might develop chronic anxiety; a child forced to hide their true identity (not understanding their sexuality due to familial or social pressure) might internalize shame that later fuels depression. These are imbalances between the individual and their environment's "terms," to paraphrase an earlier reflection. When we are in conflict with societal or developmental expectations – whether by being in a different life stage than peers, or defying social norms, or being unsupported – it generates chronic psychic stress. The brain of a young person in such turmoil is bathed in stress hormones and often deprived of consistent emotional nurturance. Over time, this shifts the calibration of systems like the HPA axis, the amygdala, and even neurotransmitter levels (for instance, chronic stress can lower serotonin and GABA). Thus, the person enters adulthood with a vulnerability: their inner balance is already tilted, like a car with misaligned wheels that's prone to skidding in rough weather.

Social context in adulthood continues to play a major role. Loneliness, discrimination, poverty, or chronic work stress can slowly grind down resilience. Humans are social creatures; feeling unsupported or marginalized is inherently stressful and can precipitate mental health issues. For instance, someone who "does not occupy the same stage of life as others" – perhaps they hit a career setback while friends advance, or they remain single while peers marry – may feel out of place. If this gap is met with self-criticism or societal judgment, it can become a source of chronic stress or depression ("what's wrong with me?" syndrome). Similarly, failing to meet family or cultural expectations – say, about career or hierarchy – can generate toxic stress. (One's place in the hierarchy does matter: studies in social mammals show that those low in rank have higher stress hormones and worse health outcomes. A lack of confidence and chronic feeling of subordination – "I am weak, I am nothing" – can drive anxiety and depression in young people, paralleling what is seen in primate hierarchies.) The point is, every life is lived in context, and that context can either buffer us or batter us. No brain exists in a vacuum, and therefore mental illness is never just "in your head" – it's usually a combination of your brain and what happened to you.

Yet, within this sobering reality lies hope: the same neuroplasticity that may have allowed bad experiences to harm you also allows good experiences and treatments to help you heal. The brain is not a static machine that simply breaks and stays broken. It's a living organ that is constantly rewiring itself based on what we do, think, and undergo. Neuroscientist Donald Hebb famously summarized neuroplasticity as "neurons that fire together, wire together," meaning if you repeatedly engage certain patterns of thinking or feeling, the connections supporting those patterns strengthen. This can cut both ways. If someone spends months or years hating themselves, trapped in self-critical thought loops, those neural pathways become deeply entrenched – a rutted road that the mind falls into by default. Chronic trauma can wire the brain to expect danger everywhere (hyper-vigilance networks wire together), and chronic despair can wire together circuits of hopelessness such that it feels impossible to imagine change. In depression, functional MRI studies have shown hyper-connectivity between certain brain regions (rumination circuits) that correlates with the uncontrollable negative thoughts patients report. In a sense, the depressive brain has learned to be depressed; it's stuck in a depressive mode that perpetuates itself via wired-in habits of thought.

But importantly, plasticity allows for new learning and unlearning. With effective therapy, for example, those rumination circuits can weaken while healthier thought patterns strengthen. This has been observed: cognitive-behavioral therapy (CBT) and other treatments can reduce overactivity in the amygdala and increase activity in the prefrontal cortex as patients learn to reinterpret fears and exert top-down control. Antidepressant medications, by boosting serotonin or other neurotransmitters, can stimulate neural growth in the hippocampus (literally recovering some volume lost to stress) and promote more flexibility in neural networks – essentially giving the brain a chance to lay down new, positive pathways. Even something as simple as exercise has been shown to increase BDNF, a growth factor, and foster new neuron formation, aiding recovery from depression. In one dramatic case, Phineas Gage – whom we met earlier – partially relearned his social skills and planning abilities over time, enough to hold a job as a stagecoach driver post-accident. His brain could not regrow the lost tissue, but it reorganized the remaining tissue to compensate, illustrating the potential for resilience and adaptation.

The idea that "once mentally ill, always ill" is outdated. The brain can heal, though the process is often slow and effortful. In fact, going through a mental health crisis and coming out the other side can sometimes lead to a state of post-traumatic growth – a deeper appreciation for life, increased empathy, and a more robust coping repertoire. Recall the earlier reflection that "anything you want will require the exact opposite. Happiness after misery. Love after heartbreak. Clarity after confusion... When things flip, you get what you want. But you have to see the other side first." There's a kernel of truth in this poetic view: experiencing the depths of misery can, in recovery, give rise to an equally profound capacity for joy and gratitude. Many recovered patients say they now feel emotions with a richness they never had before – having seen darkness, the colors of life appear more vivid. This isn't to romanticize suffering, but to highlight human resilience. The brain's plasticity is the mechanism behind this two-sided coin of experience: the very changes that led you into illness (extremes of emotion, breakdown of stability) can reverse in the presence of new experiences, new skills, and support. It's important to note, too, that not every bout of emotional suffering qualifies as a clinical disorder – and that's okay. Feeling intense grief after a loss, or anxiety during a pandemic, or demoralization in a toxic environment – these are natural responses to life's challenges. We shouldn't pathologize every struggle. A certain instability is inherent in la condition humaine (the human condition). We all go through periods of confusion, heartbreak, identity crisis. These experiences, as painful as they are, do not always mean one has a mental illness; often, they are part of the normal spectrum of life's opposites – the lows that give meaning to the highs. The difference often comes down to degree and impairment. In psychiatry, a syndrome becomes "disorder" when it causes clinically significant distress or impairment in daily functioning. In simpler terms, when the suffering is so persistent or intense that it disables you from living the life you want – holding a job, maintaining relationships, caring for yourself – then it likely qualifies as an illness that might benefit from treatment. But even short of that threshold, any suffering matters and deserves compassion. You don't need a diagnosis to seek growth or support. And conversely, getting a diagnosis should not be seen as a pigeonhole or life sentence – it's a starting point for understanding and addressing an issue.

The encouraging reality is that mental illnesses are treatable, and people do recover. There are effective prevention and treatment options for most mental health conditions, as the World Health Organization emphasizes. Therapies (talk therapies, medications, social support, lifestyle changes, etc.) can work wonders in restoring the brain's balance. Most individuals who engage in treatment see improvement, and many achieve full remission – meaning they no longer meet criteria for the disorder and can function well. Even in severe cases like schizophrenia or bipolar disorder, appropriate treatment often allows people to live meaningful lives. And beyond formal treatment, humans have a remarkable capacity for resilience – the ability to bounce back or adapt in the face of adversity. Resilience can be cultivated: through building strong relationships, finding purpose, developing coping skills (like mindfulness or problem-solving), and taking care of one's physical health (since body and mind are deeply connected). Each healthy habit or supportive connection literally strengthens neural networks that protect against stress. In essence, we can all build a buffer for our brains, making that tightrope a bit less precarious.

I write about all this not just as dry academic knowledge, but as someone who has lived it. I am a living example of how acknowledging vulnerability and seeking help can lead to recovery. I have wandered the dead-ends of depression – hating myself, losing my will to live, feeling utterly broken – and yet, with time and support, I found my way out of that maze. I've seen "the other side of the coin," and it has imbued every moment of peace and happiness now with an "intensity and appreciation that is simply impossible without seeing the other side first," to quote my past self. The brain's fragile balance tipped me into darkness, but it was also able to tip me back toward light. Each small step – talking to a therapist, taking medication as needed, confronting painful memories, rebuilding routines – helped my brain re-calibrate. It was not an overnight flip of a switch, but a gradual process of regaining stability. And it started with one pivotal act: acknowledging that I was ill and needed help. There is a profound dignity in that moment of acknowledgment. In a world that often stigmatizes mental illness, recognizing your own suffering and reaching out for aid is an act of courage. It is the first step to reclaiming balance. Just as one would not hesitate to set a broken bone, we mustn't hesitate to mend a troubled mind. By admitting "I am not okay," you affirm that you deserve to be okay – that your wellness matters. This self-honesty is the opposite of weakness; it is strength. It is the moment you stop fighting the fact of the imbalance and start fighting for your recovery. As I conclude this chapter, I want to leave you with this reassurance: mental illness is treatable, recovery is possible, and resilience is buildable. No matter how unstable things feel now, the brain can find its footing again. The journey might be long or the balance forever a bit sensitive, but you can live a fulfilling life with the right support and habits in place. Remember that every human life has its seasons of suffering – you are never alone in that – and every season changes. Accepting the sickness, giving it a name, seeking help – that is the first act of courage, the first step across the rope. From there, with patience and persistence, you can walk your way to the other side, restored to yourself with hard-won wisdom and a deeper capacity for empathy and joy.

Part II

The Major Disorders of Our Time

CHAPTER 4

The Many Faces of Addiction: The Mind's Favorite Poison

When I was growing up, a family lived in the apartment next to mine—whose shouts spoke louder than any words. I never ended up meeting the entire family in person, but I often saw Guilherme when I left for school. He would sit at the base of the stairs in the building where I spent much of my childhood. Perhaps he was already approaching old age, but it was hard to tell—his eyes carried a weight that made age seem irrelevant.

School started at 7 a.m., so I left no later than 6:30. The sun had barely risen, and there he was—hunched over, motionless, staring into nothing. One morning, when I was no older than eight, I noticed the dark circles under his eyes—so stark and swollen they looked almost like bruises. And with the kind of thoughtless innocence only a child can possess, I asked him whether someone had hit him, and if he was all right. I meant no harm—just the innocent concern of an eight-year-old. He didn't answer. I wished him a good day and ran over to my mom's car, where she was waiting to take me to school.

Clearly, my mom had seen the interaction through the windshield and she didn't look pleased. As we drove off, she told me—not unkindly, but with a tone that left no room for questions—not to bother Guilherme again. Some people, she said, prefer to be left alone. I left it at that. She hit the clutch, and we drove off to school.

Four years later, my mom told me that Guilherme had died. She had heard it from Lisa, his wife. She said it with the heaviness of someone who had long expected the news.

After living in the same building for so many years, you naturally develop a relationship with your neighbors. I had often seen Mom and Lisa chatting in the elevator, though I never paid attention to what they said. Only later in life did I connect the dots. My mom wasn't surprised by Guilherme's death—not after all the stories Lisa had shared with her in their 20-second elevator rides.

Lisa said he had disappeared five days before he was found. Apparently, that wasn't unusual. He would leave on a random Tuesday, saying he was going to grab a beer with friends. Whenever Lisa heard that, she already knew he wouldn't be coming back for days—sometimes nearly a week. No calls, no explanations. Just gone. And then, just as suddenly, he would reappear—tired, disheveled, asking only what there was to eat in the fridge. They were big topics to be shared in an elevator, but Brazilians are talkative, and quiet confessions often pass between women who've learned to carry private grief in public.

We never knew for sure what substances Guilherme used. Lisa would say that sometimes, during one of his episodes, she'd get a call from him in the middle of the night—desperate for 50 Brazilian reais. (The equivalent to less than USD $10.) He'd say it was for gas, or for food. Lisa never believed the excuses, but she feared that some dealer might be threatening him. So she always sent the money.

Even though you never had the chance to meet Guilherme, this story might not feel unfamiliar. I'm sure you've heard terrible stories about addiction—perhaps so many that they've started to blur together. These stories are important; they serve as warnings, reminders not to repeat the same mistakes. But I'm not here to lecture you on the dangers of drug use. I share this story because it illustrates something that data alone cannot convey: addiction is not abstract. It speaks through absence, silence, and the hollow routines of a life no longer lived with intention.

I'm here to show you the neurobiological mechanisms through which our brains process addiction—and to give you the freedom to do whatever you wish with that information. What exactly happens inside the brain when a person no longer feels able to stop?

There was a time, not so long ago, when addiction was spoken of only in whispers, as though naming it aloud might awaken something dangerous within us or taint the ones we love. I used to think addiction was a curse reserved for the unfortunate, the downfall of those who had strayed too far from the path of self-respect. In my household, addiction was utterly terrifying. I grew up hearing horrendous stories, imagining it tearing through my friends' lives, destroying careers and relationships. In my childish mind, addiction only happened to those who came from broken homes or had no future to look forward to.

My defensive attitude began when I was twelve, after reading the novel Vida de Droga (Life of Drugs) by Walcyr Carrasco. Never had I imagined that a required reading for school would leave such a lasting impact on my life. The book tells the story of a girl from a wealthy family who is pulled into the abyss of addiction—and never returns. That's more than enough to scare a child. But today, I'm not here to scare you. I'm also not here to reduce addiction to a syringe, a pill, or a bottle.

Addiction is not limited to the man who can no longer hold a job, or the woman who lost her children and is now scarcely recognizable to those who once loved her. It may reside in the man who pours himself another glass of wine each night—not for pleasure, but for the silence it guarantees. It may live in the woman who cannot fall asleep without the soft flicker of the television—not because the show interests her, but because the silence is unbearable. It may be found in the professional who lingers at the office long after the work is done, because home feels emptier than he can admit. And it may rest in the hands of a young girl who scrolls through images on a glowing screen late into the night—searching not for beauty or distraction, but for proof that she's still seen. It affects me. It affects you. It affects most people living on this planet today. What unites these patterns is not the object of attachment, but the mind's relationship to it.

So now, let's explore what it takes for a person to continue down a path of self-destruction—fully aware of the harm, but unable to turn back. This chapter is not written in a spirit of condemnation. I'm not here to tell you how to live your life. My aim is to offer a deeper understanding of how the brain responds to repetition, reward, and pain—and how easily those responses can shape us.

Neuroscience has shown us that the mind is plastic, ever-changing. With each repeated behavior, we carve new grooves into the brain's architecture—pathways that become roads, and roads that can turn into prisons if we stop questioning them.

The human brain is indifferent to legality or substance—it responds only to reward and repetition. Behavioral addictions, often camouflaged beneath cultural acceptance or technological convenience, are no less powerful than chemical ones. In many ways, they are more insidious, because they dress themselves in the appearance of normal life. Yes, this means exactly what you're thinking: almost anything, if abused, can become an addiction.

When I was younger, I thought I was better than people who used drugs. Deep down, there was a quiet sense of superiority that made me feel clean—and somehow stronger. In truth, it was the only thing I felt I was better at than my mother, and I clung to that with pride. Every time she lit a cigarette in front of me, I would act disgusted, boasting about how disciplined I was. It was the only moment of the day she wasn't calling me out for something I needed to fix. I never once felt tempted to try a cigarette. But I also realize now that I was never truly tested—because I never craved those substances. They weren't offered to me, or if they were, I never saw them as tempting. And not falling into temptation isn't a virtue if you never felt temptation to begin with.

It took me years to understand that the absence of visible vices does not equal the presence of virtue. I was addicted too—just to things that were easier to justify: food, screens, productivity. I turned to food when I felt overwhelmed, eating to fill the spaces I didn't yet know how to name. I was glued to my phone for hours, scrolling without purpose, chasing stimulation in tiny, flashing hits of attention. I buried myself in productivity, proud of how much I could accomplish in a day—never noticing how terrified I'd become of the emptiness that lingered in unstructured time.

At the time, none of it looked like addiction. Productivity looked like discipline. Doom-scrolling looked like typical teenage behavior. But that's the thing about addiction—it rarely looks harmful at first.

Addiction doesn't live in chemicals. It lives in behaviors, relationships, and self-image. You can be addicted to isolation—disappearing from the world whenever things get hard. You can be addicted to noise: parties, distractions, constant motion—because silence feels unsafe. You can be addicted to approval, that fleeting high of being seen and praised, even if it means performing a version of yourself that feels increasingly hollow. Even health can become addictive: gym routines, calorie counting, tracking apps, endless self-optimization. Not for vitality—but for control.

Over time, and through study and reflection, I've identified the most prevalent forms of addiction I believe are important to examine in detail. In this book, we will dive into three major obejcts of addiction: pornography, social media, and chemical substances.

The Dangers of Pornography

Pornography is one of those topics I've studied on the side for years, parallel to my professional life. Let me try to sum it all up. Up until the late 2000s – maybe 2010 at the latest – pornography was still being presented as harmless. Remember the classic "you have to know yourself" narrative? It was a message born from the sexual emancipation of women, dating back to the 1960s, especially pushed forward by progressive groups that gained traction alongside the first birth control pills. A whole generation of women reached their 40s, 50s, and 60s without ever experiencing a single orgasm. The discourse made sense at the time, especially in increasingly secular societies. But today, things are different. It's essential to recognize that there are different types of pornography, which we can categorize by the intensity of sensory stimulation – especially visuals. On one end, there's level zero: masturbation without any visual aid, relying solely on imagination. And on the other end, level ten: the heavy user, someone who spends entire days watching porn, hopping between dozens of group chats, and masturbating multiple times a day. Every day. For years.

Masturbation, as a biological behavior, is not new. Our closest primate relatives – chimpanzees, bonobos – do it. Our parents, grandparents, great-grandparents did it too. But what has changed is the frequency and intensity of visual stimulation. Before, it was a wrinkled magazine hidden under the sink, used until the pages stuck together. Or an old VHS tape, rewound and replayed a few times a week. That's a far cry from the daily, endless stream of high-definition content that exists today. Back then, life was also more active – people were thinner, hormones more balanced, physical labor more common, and most people married young and had families, which often meant more frequent sex.

Everything began to spiral when two major events collided: the spread of smartphones and the rise of fast internet. From that point on, all the dangers of porn consumption – psychological, physiological, and relational – arrived at once, concentrated in a tiny device we carry everywhere. Pornography entered the home through broadband, and suddenly it wasn't just low-resolution images or grainy clips. It was high-quality, instant-loading video: every genre, every preference, every imaginable act.

Pornography harms you in multiple ways. Hormonally, it destroys your reward system. It hijacks your brain's ability to perceive dopamine, and you get stuck in a slingshot effect, constantly chasing novelty, switching from one video to the next; not because you are enjoying them, but because you are looking for the "perfect" one to finish. You end up with forty tabs open on page 180 of a website, still searching.

Physiologically, if you are a man, your body stops responding to real women. You become conditioned to the mechanical pressure of your own hand, which exceeds anything you would experience during real sex. Your arousal patterns become dependent on the dopamine spikes from screen stimulation, which don't occur in face-to-face intimacy. This leads to erectile dysfunction – an inability to maintain an erection, and eventually the infamous "I have to finish with my hand." If you want to know if your husband is struggling with porn addiction, that's your clue: when sex always ends with him finishing alone.

Psychologically, the damage goes deeper. You lose decision-making power. You become dependent. The more you masturbate, the less capable you are of connecting sexually with another person. Imagine a man coming home from work to have sex with his wife, but he has already masturbated twice that day. And while doing so, he watched video after video of eighteen-year-old girls, gangbangs, wife swaps, violent sex, humiliation, sadomasochism. Then, after dinner, he is expected to be intimate with the woman he has been married to for twelve years, who just gave birth and has a normal adult body. It is not going to happen.

This is where it begins: avoidance. He dodges intimacy at every opportunity because his needs are already met by another source of stimulation. The symptoms of addiction begin. Real sex with his wife becomes pure frustration. And then the downward spiral begins:

He has been consuming porn daily for years. It becomes part of his routine, even if "just to sleep."

The videos become increasingly violent as his brain requires more extreme content for the same arousal.

He starts masturbating three or four times a day. Eventually, he can't even get hard – he just goes through the motions.

He stops being able to orgasm during sex. Many can't even get hard with a partner anymore. Sex becomes a source of shame and defeat. He makes excuses: "It's work," "It's the bills," "I don't know what's happening." Eventually, he just gives up.

Then comes the blame. He externalizes responsibility: "I'm not attracted to her pregnant body," "She needs to work out," "She has let herself go." At this point, the sex is over. They may still be married, but intimacy is gone.

Over time, even the videos stop working. No dopamine slingshot is strong enough. Now there's a split: some move toward gore, others toward trans content, others seek unprotected sex with prostitutes – because the more taboo, the better. Many are already taking medication just to have sex.

Finally, sex in real life ceases to exist. He now experiences sex exclusively in the third person, as a spectator. This is when wife-sharing begins, swinging, not out of kink but out of impotence. Most of these men already have hidden folders, external drives, or cloud backups with illegal content – child porn, homemade recordings with partners or relatives, often without consent. At this point, nothing available online is enough. Real sex only happens under the influence of drugs. And the truth? It has been over for a long time.

This used to be rare. You would only find men this far gone in the darkest corners – drug addicts, porn store regulars. But today? There are boys in their early twenties already in this state.

So if you ask me whether reading an erotic novel is the same as watching porn, the answer is clear: they're not even comparable. First, most erotic novels women read are just romantic stories with occasional explicit scenes. Even when sex is described, it's rarely violent. There's no dopamine slingshot effect. Reading is neurologically safe. What is the risk? Maybe, if she uses vibrators while reading and builds a routine around it, she could develop a preference for that kind of stimulation and struggle to climax without it. But without screens, daily masturbation is rare.

The real danger? When she transitions from novels to porn sites. That is when she is exposed to everything I just described for the man. In that case, my advice would be to take a more honest, less bureaucratic approach to sex. Set intentional time: nights to have dinner together, put the kids to bed early, create space to reconnect. Because it is not just about sex, it is about being together. For women, especially, it is about connection. Men, on the other hand, can often separate sex from intimacy entirely.

Let's be honest. In most marriages, this is how it plays out: life is chaotic, kids are demanding, bills are piling up, the husband isn't doing his part, and so he only seeks out his wife for sex. She is tired, overwhelmed, and says no – once, twice, five times. He gets angry. "I do everything and still get rejected." She thinks, "he only wants me for this. I'm not a doll." Meanwhile, the man wakes up in the morning wondering if tonight is "the night." He thinks about it at work, at dinner, during bedtime routines. All evening, he tiptoes, hints, reads her mood, hoping to know by midnight. And then she says, "Not tonight. I'm tired." So after an entire day of hoping, he learns, at 11:50 pm, it's not going to happen. And let's be real: many women use this "suspense" as punishment, whether because he forgot something, didn't help, didn't call his mother, or wasn't kind enough.

Now imagine this happening for months. He stops trying. But just because your husband stops trying doesn't mean he stops needing. A young, healthy man without sex will go one of two ways: porn or other women.

Now picture this: he sits down in the living room or office, opens any porn site, or logs into his OnlyFans account. The women are there, always available. That's what he turns to. He thinks, "When she wants it, she'll let me know." And she does, sure, maybe twice a month. But what about the other fifty days? He masturbates.

As porn continues to erode his ability to connect, eventually even those two times a month disappear. It is not that he does not want her anymore. It is that he cannot perform by any means. The erection fails. The intercourse has to stop halfway. He finishes with his hand. Again, again, again. Eventually, he avoids it altogether. He goes back to what's familiar: more porn.

And it is usually only at this broken point that the couple finally sees the problem. But by then, the solution is brutal: retraining desire, losing weight, quitting junk habits, seeing an endocrinologist, a nutritionist. Most men don't do it. Today, many couples in their forties have stopped having sex altogether.

And what about the woman? She feels used. Like a paid escort: paid with a house, bills, or the occasional gift. She sees a man who doesn't take care of himself, sometimes doesn't even smell clean. He drinks before sex, doesn't know how to pleasure her, doesn't treat his premature ejaculation, and is so out of shape that "sex" just means clumsily pushing a half-erect penis inside her, hoping it will work. It bends. It doesn't enter. It takes thirty minutes of oral sex to get to a halfway point – and even that is barely acceptable.

So she gives up. Especially when she's already hormonal, tired, and disconnected from her own body. Maybe she has gone through childbirth, body image issues, hormonal birth control, and now she needs the lights off, won't take off her bra, does not want to be touched. Add that to his issues? There is no sex left.

You cannot expect to have great sex without a great life. That's adolescent thinking. The reality is: when youth fades, only couples who are thriving in every area – health, finances, parenting, connection – will still have good sex. You cannot extract sex from life. That illusion dies with adulthood.

CHAPTER 5

Anxiety: The Overheated Brain

Overthinking never ends. It just keeps looping, feeding on itself and growing stronger. I know this because I've lived it – lying awake at 3 A.M. with my mind racing over every mistake I might have made, every task I should have done. Anxiety, for me, feels less like a sharp panic and more like a background hum that never switches off. It's the noise that never stops, a low-frequency dread underlying even ordinary days. In a psychology class I took at Columbia on the psychology of procrastination, I learned a striking fact: anxiety was at the core of nearly all the reasons we procrastinate. Fear of failure, fear of judgment, fear of making the wrong choice – all those fears breed avoidance. I recognized myself in that lesson. Putting off writing a paper until the night before wasn't just laziness; it was anxiety whispering "What if you do it wrong?" and luring me into delay. The cruel irony is that procrastination only amplified my anxiety, as the looming deadline grew more menacing each hour. Indeed, overthinking is the enemy we feed – an enemy fueled by the false comfort that if we just ruminate a little longer, we might gain control or certainty.

Scientifically, what's happening in an anxious brain mirrors this endless loop of worry. The brain's alarm center – the amygdala – is hyperactive, stuck in the "on" position even when no real danger is present. At the same time, the prefrontal cortex (the rational brain region that normally applies the brakes to fear) isn't doing its job well. It's as if the brain's smoke detector is hypersensitive and blaring constantly, while the firefighter in charge is half-asleep. Harvard researchers have noted this pattern: in people with anxiety, the amygdala fires off strong fear responses even to safe or neutral situations, and there's weaker connectivity to the calming prefrontal areas. In one study, patients with generalized anxiety showed higher amygdala activation than healthy people even when viewing neutral faces – essentially perceiving threat where there objectively wasn't any. After these patients underwent an 8-week mindfulness training, something remarkable happened: their brain scans showed increased connection between the amygdala and prefrontal cortex, and the amygdala stopped overreacting to neutral stimuli. In other words, by strengthening the brain's natural regulation system, the constant alarm could finally quiet down. This finding gives me hope – it suggests that the endless mental noise of anxiety isn't permanent. If the brain can learn to turn down the volume on its fear circuits, that incessant hum can fade into the background. But before we reach that hopeful note, we must first understand what lights the anxiety fire in the first place: the peculiar burdens of freedom, uncertainty, and modern life that set our minds ablaze.

The Burden of Choice and the Paralysis of Possibility

As a teenager, I believed – as many do – that I could be anything I wanted. Every door seemed open: dozens of careers, countless lifestyles, infinite versions of me. It was liberating… until it became terrifying. I remember standing at a crossroads in college, having to declare a major and feeling utterly paralyzed. Whichever path I chose meant the death of countless other lives I could have lived. I was grieving options I hadn't even lost yet. I lingered in indecision for weeks, as if keeping all possibilities open would somehow protect me. In truth, this was the illusion of control that overthinking gives us: if I endlessly consider every angle, maybe I won't have to give up anything. Of course, that's impossible – choosing something inherently means not choosing everything. I recall journaling a question to myself: "Can you stand the idea of being something instead of everything?" At 19, I honestly wasn't sure I could.

It turns out this struggle is a common development hurdle. Psychologist Erik Erikson described the adolescent task as one of resolving "identity vs. role confusion." In his theory, young people must eventually commit to an identity – a set of values, a path, a sense of self – or else remain in a morass of confusion about who they are. Erikson noted that the primary psychosocial task of adolescence is to form a coherent identity out of the many possible roles and selves one can adopt. In essence, growing up involves sacrificing possibilities to build a singular, authentic life. That realization – that I had to relinquish my dream of, say, being both a novelist and a neurosurgeon and an astronaut and a rock star, and actually pick something – hit me like a ton of bricks. It produced a kind of existential anxiety I hadn't felt before.

The existentialists understood this kind of anxiety well. The philosopher Søren Kierkegaard famously wrote, "Anxiety is the dizziness of freedom." When I first read that line, it resonated deeply. Freedom sounds wonderful until you're standing on the edge of it, looking down into an open abyss of possibilities. Then freedom feels dizzying. Kierkegaard observed that an anxious person is bewildered by their own freedom, disturbed by the fact that with every choice, they alone are responsible for the outcome. We have so many options in any situation, and nothing – except our own decision – prevents us from choosing even the most destructive path. That realization is intrinsically anxiety-provoking. A vivid metaphor Kierkegaard uses is imagining a man standing on a cliff: he's not only afraid of falling, but even more anxious that he could choose to jump. The void doesn't push him; his own freedom to leap creates the vertigo. I remember feeling a version of that vertigo when I thought about dropping out of one career path for another – the knowledge that nothing truly forced me one way or another was strangely frightening. Too many paths can feel like no path at all, leaving us stuck at the fork, frozen by the fear of regret.

Modern research backs up the idea that too much choice can breed anxiety. Psychologist Barry Schwartz dubbed it the "paradox of choice": having endless options often leads to paralysis, self-blame, and regret. With more alternatives, we find it harder to choose and easier to imagine we chose wrong. Schwartz argues that overwhelming choice overload can actually make us less happy – it feeds anxiety, stress, and even depression. I see this phenomenon every time I open Netflix and spend an hour scrolling, terrified of picking a movie I won't enjoy – a trivial decision, yet it becomes monumental in the moment. This intolerance of uncertainty lies at the heart of anxiety. We want to know we're making the right choice, that nothing better is being left on the table, but life never gives that guarantee.

In fact, some psychologists argue that uncertainty is the engine of anxiety. If fear is like a car's accelerator and reassurance the brake, uncertainty cuts the brake lines. One prominent anxiety researcher,

R. Nicholas Carleton, provocatively suggested that "fear of the unknown" might be the fundamental fear underlying all anxiety. We can tolerate a lot of known dangers, but not the nebulous what-ifs that loom in the unknown. When I procrastinate or overthink, it's often because uncertainty is gnawing at me: What if I choose wrong? What if I fail? I avoid deciding or acting, trying to postpone that uncomfortable unknown. But in doing so, I only prolong the anxiety. It's like standing in place because you're afraid the bridge might collapse – you never cross the chasm, but you never reach solid ground either.

If uncertainty is fuel for anxiety, adolescence and young adulthood provide plenty of it. Leaving the structure of childhood, we suddenly face innumerable uncertainties: Who will I become? What if I don't succeed? Whom will I love? The possibility in these questions is both exciting and terrifying. Over time, I learned (with difficulty) that one antidote to this paralysis is embracing commitment – choosing a direction and accepting the loss of alternative paths. Committing to something – a career, a relationship, a set of values – is scary, yes, but it also prunes the thicket of infinite possibilities down to a more manageable garden of choices. It reminds me of pruning a tree: it feels like a loss to cut away branches, but it ultimately allows the tree (your life) to grow taller in one clear direction. Every time I've made a hard choice and closed other doors, I've felt an initial spike in anxiety (Did I do the right thing?), followed by a gradual relief and clarity. The burden of choice lifts once the choice is made. Only then can you walk forward, lighter for having decided.

The Physiology of an Overheated Brain

What exactly is happening in the anxious brain during all this? When I describe anxiety as an ever-running motor or an overheated engine, that metaphor is surprisingly accurate to the biology. Anxiety is like the brain's fear network has been cranked up to 11 and left there. There are three major components to this "overheated" system: First, as mentioned, the amygdala – a pair of almond-shaped clusters deep in the brain – acts as the alarm system. In anxiety, the amygdala is overactivated. It's constantly sounding the alarm, even for minor triggers. Imagine a smoke detector that goes off not just for smoke, but for toast in the toaster, or even just steam from the shower. That's the anxious amygdala – hyper-vigilant, seeing danger everywhere. Brain scans across different anxiety disorders consistently show greater activity in the amygdala (and its partner-in-crime, the insula) compared to non-anxious brains. In a meta-analysis of many neuroimaging studies, patients with phobias, social anxiety, or PTSD all had this common feature: the fear centers of the brain lit up more than in healthy individuals. It's as if people with anxiety have an amygdala that's finely tuned to sniff out threat, and once it gets going, it floods the body with fear signals.

Next, the prefrontal cortex (PFC) – especially areas like the ventromedial PFC and anterior cingulate – is supposed to regulate those fear signals. If the amygdala is the accelerator, the prefrontal cortex is the brake. In anxiety, that brake often fails. Research shows that some anxiety disorders involve underactivity or inefficiency in the prefrontal cortex's control over the amygdala. For example, people with PTSD in that same meta-analysis uniquely showed lower activity in parts of the prefrontal cortex that normally help regulate emotions. In my own subjective experience, this feels like the rational part of me knows that, say, giving a presentation tomorrow isn't truly life-or-death, but it can't seem to convince my gut. The fear circuit is running hot, and the rational circuit can't cool it down. This imbalance – an overactive amygdala and an underactive regulator – is a hallmark of the anxious brain.

Then there's the HPA axis – the hypothalamic-pituitary-adrenal axis – which is our body's hormonal stress response system. When the amygdala screams "Danger!", the HPA axis releases stress hormones, notably cortisol. Cortisol is useful in actual emergencies (it helps mobilize energy and alertness), but under chronic anxiety it becomes a problem. It's like revving a car engine non-stop; eventually, parts wear out. Chronically elevated cortisol can lead to all sorts of physical symptoms: sleeplessness, racing heart, sweaty palms, tense muscles, digestive issues. I used to think it was "all in my head" until I realized it was also in my body – the headaches and knot in my stomach the night before a big exam were cortisol and adrenaline flooding my system. Research confirms that chronic anxiety keeps cortisol levels high, and that is linked to symptoms like restlessness, insomnia, a pounding heart, and sweating. Essentially, an anxious brain puts the body into a perpetual state of subtle fight-or-flight. Even when I'm sitting safely at home, my physiology might be acting as if a predator is lurking or a disaster is imminent. Over time, this wears you down. I often feel exhausted after a day of anxious thoughts, even though I've done nothing physically strenuous – it's an exhaustion from my body being on high alert for hours on end.

One vivid personal example: I used to get severe stomachaches whenever I had to have a difficult conversation or confront someone. I later learned that this was a product of my stress response – cortisol was diverting energy away from digestion (because who needs to digest lunch when you're "escaping danger"?) and that can cause gut discomfort. I was literally worrying myself sick. Chronic activation of the stress response, as one Harvard Health article put it, is like an engine idling too high for too long – eventually it starts causing damage. We know prolonged stress can contribute to high blood pressure, weakened immunity, and even changes in the brain (for example, long-term high cortisol has been linked to shrinkage in the hippocampus, a brain region important for memory). So anxiety isn't just a mental state; it's a full-body phenomenon. It's an overheated whole system.

Now, consider how this "always-on" alarm affects our social life and self-image. One thought that used to torment me in social anxiety was: "I'm burdening others". I'd worry that asking for help, or even just sharing my feelings, would weigh on my friends and family. In my anxious mind, needing others was equivalent to harming them – I feared being too much. This belief made me withdraw and avoid leaning on anyone, which ironically probably made my loved ones more worried about me. It's a common feature of social anxiety: the fear of negative evaluation, of judgment, of being an imposition. Neuroscience has shown that this fear is not just metaphorical – the amygdala, that threat detector, becomes hyperactive at the prospect of social judgment. For people with social anxiety disorder, being evaluated by others (even in something as simple as someone's facial expression or tone of voice) can trigger an amygdala alarm as intense as if they were facing actual danger\One study I read about found that individuals with high social anxiety showed greater amygdala activation when they thought they were being judged or watched. In my case, a mere "We need to talk" text from a friend could send my heart racing; my brain interpreted it as a potential social catastrophe. But here's a liberating insight I've learned: being human is to be a burden for others – and that's okay. Every relationship involves mutual burden and mutual benefit. When I was deep in anxiety, I viewed myself as a one-sided burden, imagining that any support I received was an unfair imposition on others' goodwill. Yet I never applied that standard to others when they leaned on me. In fact, helping a friend through a tough time never felt like a burden; it felt meaningful. I started to realize that my friends likely felt the same toward me. We wouldn't be in each other's lives if we didn't want to share those burdens and joys. People are adults who can make their own choices – if they choose to be close to me, they are implicitly saying, "Your problems are worth my time, as you are worth my time." Anxiety often involves a kind of arrogant overestimation of one's ability to ruin others' lives. I don't mean that harshly – I say it from having lived it. I thought if I cancelled plans or showed my sadness, I would single-handedly wreck everyone's fun. I had to remind myself: I'm not so powerful that my mere mood or request can derail someone else's entire well-being.

Social neuroscientists talk about how social pain (like rejection or negative evaluation) follows similar pathways in the brain as physical pain. No wonder it looms so large in anxiety. But we can reframe the fear. I started asking myself in anxious moments: "How am I being of service to others?" This question is a gentle prod to exit the self-preoccupation of anxiety. Instead of spiraling about how I am perceived, I try to focus on them – the person I'm with, what they might need, how I can listen or help. It's almost magical how this shifts my mindset. The amygdala quiets down when I'm not shining the spotlight on my own potential flaws. By easing up on the need to control how others see me, I also ease my brain's panic button that's tied to social approval. In effect, I'm telling my brain: It's okay if you're not perfect; you're here to connect and contribute, not to perform under scrutiny. This doesn't eliminate anxiety – I'm still a work in progress – but it turns the volume of the noise down a notch or two.

The Trap of Modern Overprotection and Self-Preoccupation

We live in an age of unprecedented self-awareness about mental health. On one hand, that's fantastic – we're finally encouraging people to talk about anxiety, depression, and stress rather than suffer in silence. But there's a paradox here. I remember writing in my journal (perhaps a bit provocatively): "The more we encourage people to be concerned about their mental state, the more good we will do… or will we? Over-focusing on oneself is definitely a path to misery." What I was grappling with is the line between healthy introspection and destructive self-absorption. Modern culture sometimes swings toward overprotection – wrapping ourselves (or our children) in bubble wrap, shielding from all adversity, encouraging constant self-check-ins for distress. The intention is compassionate, but could it be that we're inadvertently making ourselves more fragile?

There's research suggesting that overprotection can fuel anxiety. One classic finding is in parenting studies: parents who are overly protective and controlling, who shield their kids from every possible risk or failure, tend to raise children with higher anxiety levels. In a meta-analysis of 47 studies, psychologists found that parental control (the core of overprotection, meaning low autonomy given to the child) was significantly associated with greater child anxiety. Specifically, lack of autonomy – not letting kids face challenges on their own – accounted for a big chunk of the variance in whether children developed anxiety. Essentially, the less hardship you let a child encounter, the less they learn to cope, and the more anxious they become about the world. This doesn't mean we should throw children to the wolves, but it does mean that some stress inoculation is healthy.

I see parallels in adulthood. When I bubble-wrapped myself during particularly anxious periods – avoiding all triggers, saying no to opportunities out of fear, insulating myself from discomfort – my anxiety didn't get better. It often got worse. I became more sensitive to stress, not less. It's like staying in a dark room for days; when you finally step out, even normal daylight feels blinding. By contrast, when I've had structured, even challenging, routines, I've noticed my anxiety decrease. During one period, I joined a rigorous coding bootcamp (far outside my comfort zone). It was tough and stressful in a normal way – deadlines, group projects, constructive criticism. Interestingly, my general anxiety symptoms improved during those months. I had less time to ruminate and more proof each day that I could face challenges without breaking. This aligns with the idea that avoidance maintains anxiety. Psychologists often say the only way out of anxiety is through – by gradually facing the situations you fear, you teach your brain that they're survivable and not as catastrophic as the amygdala insists. Avoidance, on the other hand, is like a short-term relief (phew, I escaped that stress) that solidifies long-term fear (uh oh, I never learned that it wasn't dangerous).

We see an interesting cultural trend now: emphasizing trigger warnings, safe spaces, aversion to any discomfort. Again, the intentions are kind. But I sometimes wonder, as my journal quote alludes, if we're accidentally validating the idea that people are too fragile to handle life's bumps. A respected psychologist, Jonathan Haidt, discusses this in terms of "anti-fragility" – the notion that human beings actually grow stronger by being exposed to manageable stressors, much like our immune system strengthens through exposure to germs. When we overprotect, we deprive ourselves of the chance to build resilience. Discipline, structure, and exposure to challenges can act like a vaccine against anxiety. They aren't always pleasant in the moment (just as a vaccine shot can hurt), but they spur the growth of coping mechanisms.

I experienced this firsthand with something as simple as exercise. A few years ago, I made myself run every morning, no excuses. Initially, every fiber of my anxious brain hated it, and I felt I had to do it, which triggered my worry ("What if I miss a day? I'll beat myself up!"). But after a while, that routine became a source of stability. Rain or shine, I ran. It was a mild physical stressor that paradoxically left me mentally calmer the rest of the day. The discipline freed me from the anxiety of whether I'd exercise; it was non-negotiable, so I didn't perseverate on it. Studies have shown that predictable, repetitive routines are calming and help reduce anxiety. My morning run turned into a form of moving meditation. It also taught me that I could endure discomfort (like running in cold weather or pushing through fatigue) and be okay – a lesson directly translatable to emotional discomfort.

Another trap of self-preoccupation is that anxiety can become about itself. I've fallen into loops where I wasn't just anxious about an upcoming event, I was anxious about being anxious. It's like an echo chamber: worrying that my worry will ruin things, then worrying about the worrying – a hall of mirrors. Over-focusing on my internal state only amplified each twinge of anxiety. It's akin to picking at a wound; sometimes, leaving it alone and focusing outward heals it faster. This is why one of the most powerful shifts for me has been asking that question: How can I be of service? When I mentor a younger student, help a colleague, or even volunteer somewhere, my anxiety levels decrease for a while. Not because the underlying brain circuits magically disappear, but because I've taken the spotlight off me. The world becomes bigger than my head.

This isn't to say we should ignore our mental health – not at all. It's crucial to acknowledge and seek help for anxiety. But there's a balance between awareness and over-identification. I had to learn that I have anxiety, but I am not my anxiety. When I stopped treating myself like a fragile object and more like a capable (if occasionally struggling) person, I actually felt stronger. People around me, I realized, don't want me to suffer, but they also don't need me to be completely free of suffering for our relationships to work. In fact, sharing burdens can deepen relationships. Think of close friends who likely feel happy to support you just as you support them. Anxiety often lies to us, saying, "You're a bother, you're weak for feeling this." But consider the alternative: if a friend came to you anxious, would you see them as weak or bothersome? Of course not. You'd probably admire their courage to open up and gladly help. I had to learn to extend that same compassion to myself.

In sum, I've started to embrace a bit of tough love with my anxiety. I gently push myself to do the uncomfortable thing rather than retreat. I remind myself that life will inevitably involve being a burden at times, and that's part of the beautiful reciprocity of relationships – today you carry me, tomorrow I carry you. And crucially, I've learned that wrapping myself in psychological cotton wool only made my mind more skittish. Far better to build calluses by living, even if that means sometimes stumbling and scraping a knee. Each scrape teaches my brain that it can heal.

Value, Competition, and the Market of Life

Not long ago, I wrote in a fit of frustration: "The guy who creates more value wins… Effort alone doesn't cut it." I was reflecting on how our society often feels like a massive competition, a marketplace where human worth is measured in productivity, success, and output. Living in a big city and attending a prestigious university, I internalized the idea that I constantly had to prove my value – get the best grades, land the best internships, have the most impressive resume. The pressure was intense and, unsurprisingly, anxiety-provoking. I would attend networking events (heart hammering in my chest) feeling like I had to perform, to "sell" myself so I wouldn't fall behind my peers. There's an ambient fear that if you aren't exceptional, you'll be left behind in a brutal economic and social Darwinism.

This constant comparison – seeing colleagues publish papers, friends posting about promotions on LinkedIn, even strangers on Instagram flaunting achievements – fed a gnawing anxiety that I'm not doing enough, not being enough. Social media, especially, poured gasoline on this fire. It's like having a scoreboard of everyone's life visible at all times. When I scroll through others' highlight reels, it often triggers thoughts like, "I'm 25 and haven't done X, Y, Z yet – am I a failure?" I know rationally that social media is curated and not representative of people's full lives, but the emotional effect remains: a spike in self-doubt and worry that somehow I'm falling short.

Neuroscience offers some insight here by looking at how our brains respond to status and competition. Our brains have reward circuits (often involving the neurotransmitter dopamine) that light up when we gain something desirable – say, a promotion, or even a bunch of "likes" on a post. We can become somewhat addicted to these reward hits. Conversely, being "low status" or losing in competition registers as a threat. There's an evolutionary logic: in primate hierarchies, lower status can mean less access to resources or mates, so it's stress-inducing. Famed neurobiologist Robert Sapolsky studied baboon societies and found that an individual baboon's stress hormone levels (cortisol again) were influenced by its social rank. Generally, baboons lower in the hierarchy – who faced more harassment and uncertainty – had higher cortisol levels, indicative of chronic stress. In unstable hierarchies, even high-ranking baboons got stressed because they had to constantly fight to keep their spot. Sapolsky often draws parallels to human "rank" situations: our modern battles are not usually physical fights but battles for status, promotion, reputation. Yet our bodies react with the same primal stress response.

When I read Sapolsky's work, I had a lightbulb moment. No wonder I felt anxious at work or among my overachieving peer group – some part of my brain perceived it as a survival issue, a fight to not be the loser baboon getting pushed off the best food source. It sounds absurd in a way – no one at Columbia was literally starving or exiling me. But metaphorically, the fear is of social starvation, of being irrelevant or undervalued. That fear can drive people to work themselves to burnout. It certainly drove me to sacrifice sleep and peace of mind to get an edge wherever I could.

The trouble is, in the market of life, there is always someone producing more "value" (whatever value means – money, fame, skill). If my self-worth is tied solely to being better than others in a zero-sum sense, anxiety is guaranteed. It's like being in an endless race; even when you sprint, you see someone gaining on you. I experienced this vividly in my first job after college. I worked insane hours because

I wanted to be the top performer. I did well, but then I'd catch wind of a colleague who was published in a major outlet or who coded a brilliant program, and instantly my triumph deflated. I'd lie awake thinking, I need to do more, I'm not keeping up. My mind was perpetually in a scarcity mindset – believing that success, attention, and respect were limited resources I had to fight over.

Anxiety in this context often comes from comparisons and uncertainty about one's place. Will I succeed or will I end up "low status"? The uncertainty eats at you. Social media amplifies this with constant upward comparisons – you mostly see others' successes, rarely their struggles. A poignant example: I once posted about a professional award I got, getting likes and "congrats." What I didn't post was the months of anxiety attacks I had leading up to that project, or the imposter syndrome afterward. So I contributed to the illusion for others that I was just smoothly excelling. Realizing this made me take others' posts with a grain of salt – but still, it's hard not to feel the pang of Why not me? when scrolling.

The market mentality also skews how we view effort and reward. I wrote "effort alone doesn't cut it," which was my frustrated acknowledgment that just trying hard isn't enough; you have to produce something deemed valuable by external standards. This can be deeply demoralizing and anxiety-inducing for people (myself included) who tie their self-esteem to their outputs. If I equate my personal worth with my latest achievement, then any dip in productivity or any failure becomes a threat not just to my goals, but to my very identity. That's a lot of pressure to live under each day. So how to cope with this societal anxiety of competition? One approach I've taken is to consciously redefine what "value" means to me. Instead of defaulting to the prevailing notion (salary, awards, followers), I've tried to align it with my values (am I helping someone? Am I creating something I'm proud of? Am I growing?). Essentially, shifting from external validation to internal validation. It's not easy – the external metrics scream for attention. But I noticed that when I focus on mastery and growth rather than winning, my anxiety lessens. Suddenly it's not a deathmatch, it's a personal journey.

There's also something to be said for gratitude and sufficiency. Anxiety often focuses on what we lack and what could go wrong. Deliberately focusing on what I have and what I've done can counter that. It sounds cheesy, but listing a few things I'm grateful for (or proud of myself for) has on occasion snapped me out of an anxious tailspin about "not doing enough." It reminds me that life is not solely a ledger of wins and losses.

And let's not forget the role of inequality and real economic pressures. Some of my anxiety about competition isn't just imagined – the stakes in a capitalist society are high. Student debt, cost of living, job scarcity in certain fields – these real factors mean many of us genuinely feel we're one misstep away from financial or career ruin. That's fertile ground for anxiety. Sociologists note that eras of greater economic insecurity tend to coincide with higher prevalence of anxiety and stress disorders. It's not all in our heads; the environment matters. Recognizing this helped me feel less alone – it's not that I'm uniquely failing at coping, it's that we're swimming upstream in some stressful social currents.

Still, while I advocate for systemic changes to ease these pressures, on a personal level I had to find a way to live sanely within the system. Part of that is setting boundaries – internally and externally. Internally, a boundary that I refuse to believe I am worth less because someone else achieved something. Externally, boundaries like "no work emails after 9 PM" or taking Sundays off social media. These protect my mental real estate. When I enforce them, I notice my cortisol (and hyperactive mind) finally get a chance to settle. It's as if I step out of the race for a moment and realize the world doesn't end; in fact, it feels more spacious.

In the baboon world, interestingly, Sapolsky found that those with strong social bonds (friendships, grooming partners) had lower stress levels regardless of rank. Translating that to my life: when I foster genuine connections and a sense of community, the competitive anxiety diminishes. It's hard to feel alone on the savannah fending off rivals when you have allies by your side. I've made it a point to celebrate others' successes rather than see them as my failures. This change in mindset – from competition to coopetition or even collaboration – has been a balm. If my friend wins an award, that doesn't detract from me; if anything, it adds joy to my life because I care about them. Re-framing others' achievements as part of the richness of my social world rather than a yardstick to measure myself by is challenging (I won't lie – envy still pokes its head up), but when I manage it, it feels like breaking a spell. The tightness in my chest eases, and I can genuinely be happy for them and content with me. In summary, modern life can feel like a never-ending contest where our value is constantly under review. That can drive anxiety to a fever pitch. But by stepping back, defining our own metrics of worth, and remembering that we're all more than our CVs, we can cool the flames. I try to remind myself: I am not in a battle with my peers for existence; there is room for all of us to shine. When one person's light shines, it doesn't dim mine – in fact, it can help light the way. This mental shift is ongoing work, but it's steering me away from the frantic, scarcity-driven anxiety that once dominated my mind.

The Paradox of Discipline and Freedom

For the longest time, I had a love-hate relationship with discipline. On one hand, I craved it – I made countless schedules, self-imposed rules, aspirational morning routines. On the other hand, I rebelled against it – sometimes literally quivering at the idea of adhering to some strict regimen, as it felt like I was surrendering my free spirit. I once mused that "discipline is interesting to the extent that it can be seen as a bigger force that controls our individuality." I think what I meant was that discipline felt like an external authority, something that could steamroll my unique quirks and make me just another cog in a machine. As someone who values individuality, this was scary. I didn't want to become a rigid, color-by-numbers person defined only by duty and routine.

Yet, here's the paradox: discipline has also been my salvation from anxiety. When my life lacks any structure, when I have total freedom with no guiding rails, my anxiety tends to skyrocket. Unlimited freedom can actually feel like a curse – recall Kierkegaard's "dizziness of freedom." Absolute freedom means every decision is up for grabs, which is overwhelming. I experienced this viscerally after graduating college. For the first time, no one was structuring my time – no classes, no syllabi, no clear next steps. The world was open. I thought I'd love it, but instead I felt frozen and anxious. I slept odd hours, procrastinated on job applications, and felt vaguely purposeless. Every day I'd wake up and ask, "What am I doing with my life?" – a daunting question before I'd even had breakfast. Interestingly, once I found a job and had a daily routine again, some of that existential anxiety eased. The discipline of a work schedule, of having to be at the office at 9 AM, oddly gave me a sense of security and identity that I lacked when I was completely free-floating.

This reflects a broader truth: structured routines can reduce anxiety by adding predictability and a sense of control. When life feels too chaotic or open-ended, imposing a bit of order – even simple habits like a regular bedtime or a weekly meal plan – can be calming. Earlier I mentioned how my morning running routine helped. That's a perfect example: by making one part of my day predictable, I freed my mind from a host of anxious micro-questions (When will I exercise? Will I actually do it? What if I skip? etc.). It's like how having a stable rhythm or ritual can ground you amidst uncertainty. Many people find solace in religious or spiritual practices for this reason – there's a comforting discipline to a prayer routine or meditation practice. It's something you can hold onto when other parts of life feel unmoored.

The paradox is that discipline, which limits some freedom, can actually create a deeper feeling of freedom. When I adhere to a disciplined habit, I eventually internalize it, and it no longer feels forced – it feels like part of me. For instance, once I disciplined myself to write for 30 minutes every evening. At first it was hard (my anxious brain would rather scroll on my phone), but after a couple of months it became second nature. That routine built skill and contentment; it gave me a creative outlet and it reduced the guilt-anxiety of "I should be writing but I'm not." By constraining that half-hour for writing, I liberated myself from hours of self-flagellation and worry about not writing.

This brings to mind an existential concept: commitment. Philosophers like Sartre and Kierkegaard (each in their own way) talked about how defining oneself requires making commitments – essentially, self-imposed disciplines. Sartre famously said we are "condemned to be free," meaning we have no choice but to choose, to create ourselves through decisions. That can be anxiety-inducing (we discussed that dizziness of freedom). But Sartre also emphasized authenticity – choosing your path and then wholeheartedly committing to it, which gives life meaning. In a sense, discipline is choosing a path repeatedly, every day. It's saying, "Out of all the things I could do, I will do this." There's something peaceful about that decision, about owning it. Instead of feeling controlled by some outside force, I try to see my disciplines as expressions of my values – I control them. When I frame it that way, discipline no longer feels like an enemy of individuality, but rather its scaffold. The structure supports the building of me that I'm constructing.

However, I won't pretend this is easy or always comfortable. I still have a defiant inner child who resists when things get too regimented. If I schedule every hour of my day, part of me starts to suffocate and inevitably I'll break out with some impulsive decision (like binge-watching a show at 2 AM on a Tuesday) just to assert that I can. I've learned that balance is key. Too much freedom – chaos. Too much discipline – stifling. The sweet spot is a flexible structure. It's like jazz music: there's a basic structure and rhythm, but within that, you improvise. I try to structure the essentials (sleep, work hours, exercise, family time) and leave some buffers for spontaneity and relaxation. That way, I get the anti-anxiety benefits of routine without feeling like a prisoner of my own rules.

Another thing I discovered is that discipline in one domain can spill over positively. When I started exercising regularly (something very tangible and physical), I noticed I became more disciplined in my mental habits too – like catching myself in negative self-talk and steering toward a coping thought. It's as though proving to myself I could stick with something gave me confidence to tackle other challenges. In therapy, I once described to my counselor that I felt I had "two minds" – one chaotic and creative, one orderly and strict – and they were at war. She reframed it: maybe they can be in partnership. The creative side needs the container that the orderly side provides; the orderly side needs the vitality and joy that the creative side brings. That reframing stuck with me. It's not individuality vs. discipline as enemies, but rather individuality thriving within discipline. A garden grows wild flowers, but you still need to water it and put a fence so it's not trampled.

Even beyond the individual level, I think society reflects this paradox. We prize freedom highly (as we should), yet we also function through rules and norms. Striking the right balance is an ongoing human project. Too much authoritarian control – people suffer and anxiety comes from oppression. Too little structure – people suffer and anxiety comes from lack of safety. On a personal scale, I am my own little society trying to find equilibrium.

I'll share a concrete example of a discipline I adopted that significantly reduced my day-to-day anxiety: no phone in bed. It sounds small, but it took real discipline for a millennial like me! I realized scrolling news or social media late at night was spiking my anxiety (news is often negative, social media triggers comparison, and the blue light messed with my sleep). So I made a rule: phone on the charger away from bed at 10 PM, and I would read a book for 30 minutes before sleep instead. The first week was brutal – I had FOMO and restlessness. But soon it became a cherished ritual. I found my sleep improved, I had fewer racing thoughts at night, and I actually looked forward to my reading time. This disciplined cutoff created a peaceful boundary around my mind at night. I share this to illustrate how a seemingly strict rule (no phone after 10) translated into more mental freedom (free from information overload and late-night anxiety).

Ultimately, I'm learning that true freedom is not the absence of constraints, but the choice of the right constraints. By consciously choosing some limits – be it a waking time, or a commitment to honesty, or a creative practice – I paradoxically feel more free from the whims of anxiety and distraction. Discipline gives me traction in life; without it I was spinning wheels, which is a very anxious feeling. Now, when anxiety flares, I actually lean on my disciplined habits to carry me through the storm: Just do your routine, trust it. In those moments, I'm grateful that past me installed some guardrails.

In closing this section, I have to smile at my younger self who thought discipline was the death of individuality. I now see it as the backbone that allows individuality to stand upright. My quirks, my spontaneity, my creativity – they all flourish more brightly against a backdrop of stability that I cultivate through discipline. The paradox resolved itself in practice: by being a little rigid, I become more relaxed. And for an anxious soul, relaxed moments are pure gold.

From Fire to Light

Anxiety has been the through-line of everything I've discussed – the endless overthinking, the paralysis of too much freedom, the racing heart and restless nights, the striving and comparing, the yearning for structure. At times, my anxiety has felt like a wildfire raging through my mind: uncontrollable, consuming, destructive. It burned hot and left me scorched with exhaustion. But as I've navigated this journey, I've come to realize that this same fire, under control, can also be a source of light.

By "light," I mean insight, empathy, even motivation. Anxiety is, in a twisted way, a form of caring – caring deeply about outcomes, about others, about doing right. The dial is just turned up too high. If I can lower the flame to a steady glow, that care becomes a positive guiding light. For example, because I've felt intense anxiety, I've also developed a profound compassion for others who suffer. It's made me more attuned to when someone else is uncomfortable or afraid, and I find myself using my hard-won coping tools to comfort them. My anxiety fire, when managed, fuels a warmth in me – a desire to help, to connect. In that sense, anxiety has shaped me into a more thoughtful and empathetic person. That's a light I wouldn't want to extinguish.

Nearly 1 in 3 people will experience an anxiety disorder in their lifetime, so I know I'm far from alone in these struggles. Anxiety is a deeply human experience, tied into our very evolution and survival.

A brain that can envision the future (a miraculous thing) also envisions possible threats (the double-edged sword). If I've learned anything, it's that I need not view my anxiety as a monster to be slain, but as a fire to be understood. Sometimes it rages out of control – then I must call on every tool (therapy, medication, meditation, support from loved ones, discipline, perspective) to tame it. But sometimes, that fire is a signal or a protector, and I can listen: What's making you afraid? Is there a real issue here to address? In those moments, anxiety illuminates something important to me – a value, a unresolved trauma, a change I need to make. It's showing me where my heart and mind are engaged.

The culture of over-choice and hyper-competition we live in throws plenty of logs on the anxiety fire. Recognizing that helps – it's not that I'm simply "weak" for feeling this way; there are real flames out there to contend with. But through personal reflection and the science we've explored, I've gained a toolkit and, critically, hope. I've seen that the brain can change (like those mindfulness practitioners whose amygdalae quieted down). I've experienced that life circumstances can change – uncertainty can resolve, choices can be made, new structures can form – and with them, anxiety can recede. And I've felt pride that I can endure anxiety's heat and still move forward.

An analogy I use now is that of a steam engine. In old locomotives, you have a fire burning to create steam that drives the engine. Anxiety, to me, is like that fire. Unchecked, it can blow the whole engine; but tended carefully, it can generate forward momentum. I try to take the energy anxiety gives (because let's face it, anxiety is energizing, just not always in a pleasant way) and channel it. Before a presentation, I'll tell myself, "This adrenaline is my body giving me fuel to perform well," rather than, "Oh no, I'm panicking." Reframing anxiety as excitement or as motivation doesn't always work, but when it does, I truly turn that fire into light – into something useful.

As I conclude this chapter of reflection, I'm aware that anxiety is only one side of the coin. There's another mental state I've known, almost the polar opposite: depression. If anxiety is an overactive brain (fire everywhere), depression can feel like the ashes after the fire has burned out – a cold, gray heaviness where nothing sparks joy. In my life, I've sometimes swung from anxious frenzy to depressive shutdown. It's as if after so much sustained worry, the mind and body say, "I can't anymore," and numbness takes over. Where anxiety is fear of the future, depression can be resignation about the future. They are different beasts, yet they intertwine (many people, including me, have experienced them as two sides of a coin). I mention this because moving forward, it's important to explore that landscape of depression – the darkness that sometimes follows when the anxious flames die down and leave one in emptiness.

For now, though, I want to leave on a note of resilience. The journey through anxiety has shown me that I'm capable of far more than I once thought. Every time I thought, "I can't handle this," I eventually did – maybe not perfectly, maybe with some tears and sleepless nights, but I came out the other side. If anxiety is the enemy we feed, we can also learn to starve it of its worst food (avoidance, isolation, self-criticism) and instead feed ourselves with better things (facing fears step by step, connection, and self-compassion). In doing so, the enemy can sometimes become an uneasy ally – a source of vigilance that, kept in check, helps me navigate life's perils with caution but not panic.

The noise in my head may never be completely silent – and that's okay. I've made peace with the idea that a certain hum of worry might just be part of my temperament. Rather than fighting it, I tune it like one might tune background music: low enough that I can focus on the melody of life in the foreground. And when the volume spikes, I now have my repertoire of strategies to turn it down. I'm turning what was once a raging fire into a steady light by which I can see and grow. In the next part of this journey, I'll delve into that realm of depression – the aftermath of the fire, the quiet darkness that can settle in. If anxiety kept me sprinting through a maze of worries, depression was like finding myself at a dead-end, too weary to retrace my steps. But just as we've seen with anxiety, there is understanding to be found there, and eventually, a path through. For every fire that burns out, dawn's light eventually comes. Let's move from the fire into the light of a new understanding, carrying forward the lessons anxiety taught, and ready to confront the shadows of despair with the same honesty and hope.

From fire to light – that is the journey. And I am still on it, step by step, day by day, turning the embers of anxious struggle into the glow of insight and strength for the road ahead.

CHAPTER 6

Depression: The Silent Void of Sadness and Suicide

The Weight of the Darkness

I wake up and immediately wish I hadn't. The morning light creeping through the blinds brings no warmth – only a reminder that I have to face another day I feel utterly unprepared for. My chest is heavy, as if I've been carrying an invisible weight through the night. Simple tasks like getting out of bed or brushing my teeth feel herculean. There's no dramatic wailing or visible wound; instead, there's a hollow numbness that has settled in my bones. I move through the motions of life on autopilot, exhausted by a battle raging silently in my mind. At my lowest point, I remember sitting on the edge of my bed past midnight, tears streaming down without sound, contemplating whether being alive was worth the pain. It wasn't that I wanted to die – I only wanted an escape from the relentless ache inside. In those anguished moments, the idea of ending it all felt like a perverse kind of relief, a final quietus to the inner turmoil. This is what depression brought me to: a place where even suicide could masquerade as a friend.

A lonely figure sitting in darkness, head in hands – a stark visual metaphor of the isolation and pain that depression inflicts. In the depths of depression, one can feel utterly alone in a world drained of color and warmth.

Depression isn't just sadness or having a bad day. It is a totalizing void that swallows joy, hope, and energy. On the outside, I often managed a weak smile; on the inside, I felt dead and disconnected. Nothing interested me anymore – hobbies, friends, even the foods I loved tasted like ash. As the existential psychologist Rollo May once wrote, "Depression is the inability to construct a future." When you're depressed, tomorrow seems empty of any promise, and next week feels impossible. In my darkest periods, I couldn't envision any future for myself at all – not even a bleak one. It was as if my life was a book that had abruptly lost its plot; every direction looked like a dead end. This illness brings a profound hopelessness about what lies ahead, convincing you that things will never get better. I wasn't alone in feeling this way. Clinical descriptions of depression note that persistent hopelessness, low self-worth, guilt, and even thoughts of death are common symptoms. Depression takes over both mind and body: I either slept for 14 hours or not at all; some days I couldn't eat, other days I binged without pleasure. I felt tired all the time, yet rest never refreshed me. My limbs were leaden, movements slow. Concentration shattered – reading a single page or following a simple conversation was a struggle. Perhaps worst of all, depression flooded my thoughts with relentless self-criticism: every mistake from my past played on loop, convincing me I was worthless and undeserving of love. This lie that my brain told – that I was utterly alone, broken, and beyond help – felt so real that I believed it.

I learned that depression lies. It whispered that no one cared, even when loved ones tried to reach me. It told me I was weak and "should just snap out of it," echoing the stigma I'd heard in society. In truth, depression is a mental disorder – a medical illness – not a personal failing. Millions of people have felt what I was feeling. In fact, depression is extremely common and widespread. According to the World Health Organization, it's now the leading cause of ill health and disability worldwide. By 2017, over 300 million people around the globe were living with depression, and that number has only grown since. The most recent estimates indicate roughly 332 million people suffer from depression worldwide – about one in every 20 people on the planet at any given time. To put it another way, around 5–6% of all adults are experiencing depression as we speak, with women about 1.5 times more likely to be affected than men. Over the course of a lifetime, the odds of encountering this illness at least once are even higher – roughly one in six of us will experience a major depressive episode in our lifetime. These numbers are staggering, yet behind each statistic is a human story like mine: someone struggling silently under the weight of an invisible pain.

Given how pervasive it is, depression has enormous human and societal costs. It doesn't just make people feel miserable – it can cripple one's ability to function day to day. It's common for depression to interfere with work, studies, and relationships. The simplest chores go undone; personal hygiene can deteriorate; social interactions become daunting or are avoided altogether. I remember the piles of unopened mail and unwashed dishes that accumulated as I battled just to survive each day. The world shrinks when you're depressed: my bedroom became both a sanctuary and a prison. Phone calls from friends went unanswered for weeks. I skipped family gatherings with flimsy excuses, because I could not bear to pretend I was okay. Unfortunately, this withdrawal and isolation often make the depression even worse, creating a vicious cycle. The stigma surrounding mental illness doesn't help either – I was afraid to tell most people how I felt, worrying they'd think I was "crazy" or weak. This is a common experience; many with depression hide their pain.

The WHO noted that prejudice and misunderstanding about mental illness stop people from seeking help, which is why their campaign slogan became "Depression: let's talk." As one WHO director put it, talking to someone trustworthy is often the first step to healing. Breaking that silence is hard, but so important.

When Darkness Deepens: Depression and Suicide

Untreated and unaddressed, depression can deepen into despair, and for some, that despair can become life-threatening. A harrowing truth about depression is that it can lead to thoughts of suicide – and sometimes suicide attempts – as people desperately seek relief from unbearable pain. Suicide is not some rare occurrence of the very few; it's tragically common. In 2021 alone, an estimated 727,000 people lost their lives to suicide around the world. Think about that: nearly three-quarters of a million souls gone in one year – more than the population of many entire cities – due to suicide. It is one of the leading causes of death in young people in particular. Globally, suicide now ranks among the top causes of death for teenagers and young adults. According to WHO data, suicide was the third leading cause of death among 15–29-year-olds in recent years (only accidents and violence typically rank higher). This means that in virtually every country, we are losing young lives to suicide at an alarming rate. And depression is a major driving factor in those suicides.

Why would a person consider such a drastic, final act? From the outside, suicide often seems incomprehensible or "selfish" to those who haven't experienced that level of despair. But I can tell you, from having stood on that abyss's edge, that the mind in a suicidal depression is not thinking rationally – it's overwhelmed by pain. "People who die by suicide don't want to end their life; they want to end their pain." I don't remember where I first heard that quote, but it rings absolutely true. When I thought about ending my life, it wasn't because I hated life itself; it was because I felt trapped in agony with no other way out. Depression had convinced me that my future would be nothing but this same pain repeating endlessly. In that distorted state, death starts to look like the only door out of a burning building. It's a lie – a deadly lie – that the depressed brain tells: that your pain will never ease and that you are a burden on others. I believed that lie. I genuinely thought my family and friends would be better off without me around to "drag them down." These kinds of thoughts are actually symptoms of the illness – the hopelessness, the self-loathing, the warped belief that your death might be a relief to others – all are cruel tricks depression plays on the mind.

To others reading this: if you have ever felt this way, know that you are not seeing things clearly while in that state. Depression places a dark filter over reality, making the good seem invisible and the bad seem insurmountable. In those moments, I wish I had known that my mind was lying to me. I wish I could have seen that my loved ones would have been devastated to lose me, that help was available, and that life could feel worth living again someday. But depression can be blinding. It can also be very convincing in its nihilism – philosophers have recognized this. The writer Albert Camus famously said "There is only one really serious philosophical problem, and that is suicide." In The Myth of Sisyphus, Camus opens by arguing that the fundamental question of life is whether to continue living or not – whether life has meaning enough to justify enduring suffering. That resonates with how one feels in deep depression: you are forced to confront, in a raw way, the question of whether life is worth all this pain. Camus ultimately concluded that even though life can feel absurd and devoid of meaning, ending it solves nothing – "there can be no more meaning in death than there is in life," he wrote. In other words, if life feels meaningless, cutting it short won't magically produce meaning; it only ends your ability to ever find meaning.

At the time I first read Camus, his words felt cold comfort – I wasn't sure I agreed with him that life's absurdity should be embraced with a smile. When you are hurting that much, high philosophy can feel disconnected from your reality. And yet, there is a kernel of truth in it: suicide is a permanent solution to a temporary problem, as the saying goes. If I had gone through with it on one of those terrible nights, I would have snuffed out any chance of things ever improving. I would have transferred my pain to the hearts of everyone who cares about me (a fact I failed to fully grasp at the time). It's an understatement to say I'm glad I didn't go through with it. Life did get better. It took time, and help, and a lot of hard work – but the darkness did recede. I lived to see days when I genuinely felt joy and peace again, emotions utterly unimaginable to me during the worst of the depression. I was fortunate; I received treatment and support in time. Many others, sadly, do not get that chance. That's why we must talk openly about suicide – to reach those who are suffering in silence and help them see that there are other ways to end their pain besides ending their life.

Understanding the Beast: What Depression Really Is

What exactly is happening to someone going through major depression? For something so common, depression is often deeply misunderstood. It's not a character flaw, laziness, or simply a bad attitude. Depression is a medical condition with well-defined features. Doctors diagnose it based on specific signs and symptoms. These include a persistently low or irritable mood, loss of interest or pleasure in activities (what used to be called "anhedonia"), significant changes in sleep and appetite, low energy, poor concentration, feelings of worthlessness or excessive guilt, and recurrent thoughts of death or suicide. To meet the clinical definition, several of these symptoms must be present nearly every day for at least two weeks and cause significant distress or impairment in functioning. In my case, I ticked nearly every box on that list.

It's important to emphasize that depression is not just intense sadness. Sadness is a normal human emotion that comes and goes in response to life events. Depression, by contrast, can arise even when everything in life seems "fine." It tends to blunt all emotions, not just happiness – many depressed people feel not only sad, but also numb or empty. I often describe it as feeling like a dark grey cloud settled over my mind and heart, dulling everything. Things that should make you laugh or smile don't have an effect. Things that would normally upset you might not even elicit tears, because nothing really sparks feeling anymore. It's like your emotional circuits short out under the overload of hopelessness. And depression isn't simply grief either – grief is painful, but typically it comes in waves and remains connected to the loss of something specific. Depression can feel like grief without a focus, sorrow without a name, a mourning of oneself and life in general.

Scientists and doctors now understand depression as a complex interplay of factors in the brain and body. There is no single cause of depression. Instead, research indicates that depression results from a combination of biological, psychological, and social factors. In other words, your brain chemistry, your genetic inheritance, your personality style, and the stressful or traumatic events you've experienced can all contribute to the development of depression. This is known as the "bio-psycho-social" model of mental illness. In my case, I can identify several risk factors: depression runs in my family (suggesting a genetic predisposition), and I went through some adverse life events that likely triggered my episode – including losing my job and a close friend in the same year. People who endure abuse, severe loss, violence, or extreme stress have a higher chance of becoming depressed. Chronic pressures like poverty or an unstable home environment can also grind a person down over time. And sometimes, depression seems to strike out of nowhere, even in a life that outwardly appears "good" – a reminder that this illness does not discriminate.

A lot of people assume depression is caused purely by a "chemical imbalance" in the brain – you've probably heard the explanation that depression is due to low serotonin levels or something similar. For many years, the serotonin hypothesis (the idea that depressed people just have deficient serotonin, one of the neurotransmitters that affect mood) was very popular. It's an appealingly simple story – take a pill to boost serotonin, fix the depression – but reality is far more nuanced. In fact, recent scientific reviews have found no clear evidence that low serotonin is the primary cause of depression. A comprehensive analysis in 2022 concluded "there is no convincing evidence that depression is caused by serotonin abnormalities, particularly lower levels or reduced activity of serotonin." This doesn't mean that brain chemistry doesn't play a role – it certainly does – but it means our earlier over-simplified explanation was incomplete. Antidepressant medications (like SSRIs) do affect serotonin, and many people feel better on them, but scientists now think these drugs may work through more complex downstream effects on brain circuits and growth factors rather than merely "correcting" a chemical imbalance. The truth is that depression's biology is multifaceted: it involves subtle changes in brain networks, stress hormones, immune system activity, and more. For instance, brain imaging studies have found differences in certain brain regions (like the amygdala and prefrontal cortex) in people with depression, especially when processing emotions. Prolonged depression is also linked to increased inflammation in the body and higher levels of the stress hormone cortisol. There's even evidence that severe stress or trauma can physically shrink parts of the brain (like the hippocampus, which is involved in mood regulation and memory) – but the good news is, effective treatment and recovery can potentially reverse these changes over time.

So, depression often arises from a tangle of genetics, brain chemistry, life experiences, and personality. If you have a family history of depression, you're at greater risk. If you tend toward pessimistic or self-critical thinking patterns, that can also make you more vulnerable. And certainly, major life stresses or trauma can precipitate a depressive episode. My own depression felt like the cumulation of long-building stress, unresolved grief, and likely some biological predisposition I never asked for. One thing I had to learn was that depression was not my fault. You can do everything "right" in life and still get depression, just as one can still get diabetes or asthma. Telling someone with depression to "just cheer up" or "try thinking positive" is as futile as telling someone with asthma during an attack to "just breathe, it's not that hard." The internal processes of depression are not under simple voluntary control; it's a health condition that requires understanding and care.

Interestingly, depression is often interconnected with other health issues. It rarely exists in a vacuum. For example, depression can both contribute to and result from substance abuse problems. Some people, in an attempt to numb their emotional pain, turn to alcohol or drugs – I admit, I drank heavily for a few months as a misguided form of self-medication. This can spiral into addiction, which then deepens the depression, forming a destructive feedback loop. Health experts have observed strong links between depression and other disorders: depression increases the risk of developing a substance use disorder, and conversely, having an addiction or chronic illness raises your risk of becoming depressed. Similarly, depression often goes hand in hand with anxiety – in fact, about half of people with depression also experience significant anxiety symptoms. I experienced this too: even as I felt numb and hopeless, I was also constantly on edge, worrying about everything and nothing. It's as if my mind was stuck in a tragic paradox – simultaneously too numb to enjoy life and too anxious to relax.

Seeking Meaning Amidst Suffering

When you're in the throes of depression, it can feel like meaning and purpose have vanished from your life. One of the hallmark thoughts of depression is "What's the point of anything?" I asked that question endlessly in my journal entries. I wrote bleak, one-line summaries like "Another day, nothing feels worth it." Philosophers, theologians, and writers throughout history have grappled with this existential void. Is there meaning in suffering? Is there any reason to keep going when every day is painful? These questions lie at the heart of both depression and the human condition itself.

One person whose reflections helped me was Viktor E. Frankl, a psychiatrist and Holocaust survivor. Frankl endured unimaginable suffering in Nazi concentration camps, yet he emerged with a powerful perspective on how humans cope with pain. In his famous book Man's Search for Meaning, Frankl argues that even when we face suffering that we cannot change, we retain the freedom to choose how we respond to it. He observed that those prisoners in the camps who found some meaning – whether a loved one to live for, or a project, or even just a decision to face suffering with dignity – were more likely to survive. Frankl wrote, "A man who becomes conscious of the responsibility he bears toward a human being who affectionately waits for him, or to an unfinished work, will never be able to throw away his life. He knows the 'why' for his existence, and will be able to bear almost any 'how.'" In other words, finding a "why" – a reason to live, no matter how small – can carry us through the darkest of times. When I first read that line, it moved me to tears. I realized I did have a why: my younger sister, who looked up to me; my dog, who would have wondered why I never came home; the book I always dreamed of writing. These were small sparks of meaning that depression had obscured but not extinguished. Frankl's words reminded me that even if life objectively seemed pointless in the moment, I could choose to pursue tiny purposes – like surviving one more day just to see what happens, or living not for myself (since I didn't value myself then) but for those who cared about me. Clinging to those threads of meaning was crucial. It didn't instantly cure my depression, but it gave me something to hold onto in the storm – a lifeline made of purpose.

Frankl also said, "If there is a meaning in life at all, then there must be a meaning in suffering." That's a challenging statement – and not everyone will agree – but I interpret it as this: our pain can shape us and push us to grow, if we let it. Suffering for its own sake is not inherently ennobling, of course. Yet, as I slowly recovered, I found that my depression fundamentally changed me, in some surprising positive ways. It broke me down, yes – but in putting myself back together, I developed a deeper empathy for others in pain, and a greater appreciation for the good moments in life. In a strange way, depression made me more human – it forced me to confront big questions and ultimately helped me redefine my values. I would never romanticize depression; if I could have avoided that hellish experience entirely, I would have. But having gone through it, I can choose to extract meaning from it. I now volunteer at a crisis hotline, something I likely would never have done had I not known what suicidal despair feels like. That gives my past suffering at least a glimmer of purpose – it equipped me to help someone else. This is the sort of transformation Frankl alludes to: turning personal tragedy into triumph not by erasing the pain but by using it for something good.

Another philosophical perspective that resonated with me is the concept of the "Absurd hero" from Camus. Camus believed that even in a life that might have no ultimate meaning, we can choose to live fully and defiantly in spite of – or because of – that absurdity. He famously concluded his essay on the mythological figure Sisyphus (condemned to roll a boulder up a hill for eternity) by saying, "One must imagine Sisyphus happy." Camus suggests that we can be like Sisyphus: aware of life's struggles and lack of clear meaning, yet not giving in to despair. Instead, we embrace life as it is, find our own meanings (like Sisyphus possibly finding meaning in the act of pushing the boulder itself), and thereby triumph over the absurd by continuing on. In the depths of my depression, thinking of myself as an "absurd hero" in Camus's sense actually brought a wry smile to my face. If nothing inherently mattered, I figured, I was free to create my own tiny missions. One mission became: "Let me survive today." Another: "I'll take care of my dog, because to her, I am the whole world." These almost absurdly small goals kept me tethered to life. They were my revolt against the nihilism that depression whispered.

From Darkness to Dawn: Finding Help and Hope

For a long time, I thought I had to battle depression alone – partly out of shame and partly out of the belief that nothing and no one could help me. I was so wrong. Help is available, and depression is treatable. In fact, mental health professionals consider depression one of the most treatable mental illnesses. There are several effective approaches, and often a combination works best. In my case, the turning point was finally confiding in someone and seeking professional therapy. I still remember the day I truly opened up to a close friend about what I was going through. Instead of the judgment and awkwardness I feared, I was met with compassion – and an insistence that I didn't have to suffer alone. With their encouragement, I booked an appointment with a therapist. I started on the road to recovery the day I walked into that therapist's office, shaking and skeptical, but desperate for relief.

Treatment for depression typically comes in a few forms (sometimes used together): psychotherapy, medication, and lifestyle changes. Therapy gave me a safe space to untangle the knotted thoughts in my head. One evidence-based form, Cognitive Behavioral Therapy (CBT), taught me how to catch and challenge the negative thought patterns depression had established. For example, when my mind would scream "you're worthless," I learned to respond, "that's the depression talking – what's the evidence for that claim?" Bit by bit, I built mental habits that countered the self-critical lies. Therapy also helped me process the grief and trauma that had fueled my depression, under the guidance of someone who understood this illness deeply.

I also decided, after consultation with a psychiatrist, to try antidepressant medication. I was initially hesitant – partly due to the stigma ("Does needing an antidepressant mean I'm really crazy or weak?" I worried) and partly due to fear of side effects. But the doctor explained that antidepressants are a legitimate tool that help millions; needing one is no more shameful than a diabetic needing insulin. The first medication I tried (an SSRI) took about six weeks to kick in. It wasn't a night-and-day difference, but one day I noticed that the constant dark cloud had lifted just a little. The edges of things were less bleak. The medication wasn't a happy pill – it didn't make me giddy or artificially cheerful – it simply raised the floor of my mood enough for the other parts of therapy and life to start helping. For some people, therapy alone might be sufficient; for others, medication provides the biochemical boost needed to restore balance. There is effective treatment for mild, moderate, and severe depression alike – it's all about finding the right approach for the individual. In more severe or resistant cases, treatments like ECT (electroconvulsive therapy) or newer interventions (like ketamine infusions or TMS – transcranial magnetic stimulation) can be considered. ECT, despite its scary Hollywood image, is a well-studied procedure done under anesthesia that can rapidly help severe depression that hasn't responded to anything else. Meanwhile, promising research in recent years has explored the use of psychedelic-assisted therapy (with substances like psilocybin) for depression, yielding some remarkable results in clinical trials – though this is still an emerging area. The landscape of treatment is expanding, and there is real, documented hope for even the most stubborn depressions.

It's also crucial to mention the little things that helped me climb out of the hole. Depression often saps our routine and self-care, so a big part of recovery was gradually reintroducing healthy habits. Simple stuff like forcing myself to take a walk each morning, even if I only managed 10 minutes at first. There were days I shuffled like a zombie through the neighborhood, head down – but the fresh air and movement, though subtle, had a cumulative effect. Exercise, even gentle, is known to have antidepressant benefits by releasing endorphins and promoting neural growth. I began paying more attention to my sleep schedule, since erratic sleep was both a cause and effect of my mood downturns. I cut back on alcohol once I realized it was a depressant drug that made my lows even lower. Instead, I tried to drink more water and eat regular, balanced meals (depression had caused me either to skip meals or overindulge in comfort food; both extremes left me feeling worse physically). None of these lifestyle changes were magic cures, but each was like a tiny brick in the foundation of recovery.

One of the hardest but most rewarding steps was reconnecting with people. Depression made me want to crawl under a rock away from everyone. But isolation is both what depression craves and what it feeds on. By reaching out – whether texting an old friend, joining a support group, or simply sitting with family in the living room even if I felt withdrawn – I began to rejoin the world of the living. Human connection is salve for a wounded mind. I vividly recall attending my first depression support group meeting: sitting in a circle of strangers, hearing my feelings come out of their mouths, was eye-opening. I wasn't uniquely broken after all; there were others who truly understood the emptiness and yet were fighting to get better, just like me. It forged a sense of camaraderie and hope that I had been missing.

There is an African proverb that says, "When you pray, move your feet." For me, moving my feet – taking those action steps – was prayer in motion, a sign that some part of me still believed in the possibility of change. And slowly, change did come. I'll never forget the morning I stepped outside and noticed the birds singing – truly noticed them – for the first time in ages. Or the afternoon I found myself laughing at a joke, and then surprised (as if, Wait, laughter? Where did that come from?). These small moments were evidence that the real me was still in there, not lost forever. Piece by piece, I rebuilt my life from the rubble that depression had left. It wasn't a neat, linear process. I had setbacks – nights when the suicidal thoughts crept back in, days when the heaviness returned out of nowhere. But each time, I had more tools at my disposal to cope. I had a therapist to call, friends to lean on, techniques to try. I learned to ride out the waves rather than drown in them.

As I write this now, I wish I could send a message back in time to the version of me that felt worthless and doomed. I would tell that younger self: Hold on. You are needed, you are loved, and you will find happiness again. If you, dear reader, are in that dark place, consider this chapter a message in a bottle from someone who made it through. You are not alone. Millions fight the same fight every day, and many of us make it to calmer seas. There is no shame in having depression – it doesn't mean you're weak or broken, it means you're human and you're hurting. It's okay to seek help; in fact, it's brave. Talk to someone you trust about how you feel. See a doctor or counselor if you can. If the burden feels unbearable, reach out to crisis resources; there are compassionate people ready to help you 24/7. The thing about depression is, it lies – it convinces you that there's no hope, but in reality, there is hope even when you can't feel it.

Life After Depression: A New Dawn

Recovering from a major depression was one of the hardest things I've ever done. But on the other side of it, life tastes sweet again. I appreciate the smallest things now – a warm cup of coffee in the morning sunlight, or the sound of my niece's laughter – in a way I never did before depression. It's as if having seen life in greyscale, I now cherish every bit of color. I won't pretend that I'm "depression-proof" going forward. Mental health can be a lifelong journey, and I still have to be mindful of my stress and emotional well-being. I know the symptoms to watch out for, and I've built a toolbox of strategies to hopefully prevent a relapse. But even if depression ever knocks on my door again, I am no longer afraid of it. I know it can be fought, and I know I'm not fighting alone.

Looking at the bigger picture, it's clear that as a society we have a lot of work to do regarding depression and mental health. On a global scale, the majority of people with depression still do not receive adequate treatment. In high-income countries like mine, an estimated 50% of people with depression go untreated; in low- and middle-income countries, a staggering 75–85% receive no treatment at all. This can be due to lack of mental health services, cost barriers, or the lingering stigma that makes people avoid seeking help. We must change this. Depression is not a moral weakness; it's a health issue that deserves the same attention and resources as any other serious illness. Every country, every community should treat mental health as a priority – because the cost of inaction is measured in lost productivity, broken families, and tragically, lost lives. The economic burden of depression (in terms of healthcare costs and lost productivity) is immense, running into hundreds of billions of dollars globally, but the human cost is beyond measure. On the positive side, investing in mental health pays dividends. The WHO has noted that every dollar spent on scaling up treatment for depression and anxiety leads to about a $4 return in better health and ability to work. More importantly, it leads to people regaining their lives. I am one of those people – someone who went from barely functioning to contributing to society again, thanks to treatment.

So, what can we do? We can start by talking openly about depression, just as we would about diabetes or cancer. This helps erode stigma and lets those who suffer know they aren't alone or weird. We can educate ourselves and others that depression is a real illness caused by real factors, and that it's not something you can just "snap out of." We can push for better access to mental health care – like integrating mental health services into primary healthcare, so that when you visit a family doctor they also check on your psychological well-being. We can support community programs and school-based initiatives that teach coping skills and emotional resilience, which have been shown to help prevent depression in young people. Even encouraging basic healthy habits in society – exercise, good nutrition, social connection – can make a dent, since these help protect against depression to some extent. On an individual level, being there for friends or family who might be struggling makes a huge difference. Sometimes just having one person to confide in can be life-saving.

I often think of the Japanese art of Kintsugi, where broken pottery is repaired with gold. The idea is that the piece is more beautiful for having been broken. I won't claim I'm more beautiful for having had depression, but I do feel… renewed. I have cracks and scars, yes, but they are filled with hard-won wisdom, compassion, and strength. I feel a kinship with anyone who has fought this fight. We are all survivors of something. If you are still in the battle, please stay. The world needs you here, even if your depressed mind tells you otherwise.

To end, I want to return to the personal – because this chapter began with my individual story, but it's echoed by countless others. Depression brought me to my knees and nearly convinced me to end my life. But with help, I gradually stood up again. And in rising, I found that the world, though imperfect, holds unexpected joys and meanings I would have missed had I checked out early. Dawn eventually came, and it was breathtaking. I step outside now and feel the sun on my face with a gratitude that only someone who has shivered through a long, dark night can feel. Life is worth living. That's something I couldn't say and believe a few years ago; now I say it with conviction. If you're in darkness, hold on – dawn is coming for you too. And when it arrives, you'll be so glad you're here to see it.

Part III

Forces Driving the Collapse

Chapter 7

Cancel Culture and Negativity

Freedom and the Death of Dialogue

Freedom means being able to do anything that does not infringe on the freedom of another. If I discriminate against someone or act on prejudice (be it racial, gender-based, or class-based), I violate someone else's freedom. In doing so, I forfeit my own freedom to that extent. Those are not the cases we're discussing here. We're talking about people who are cancelled for being free – that is, for expressing themselves in a way that doesn't actually violate anyone else's rights. These are individuals who spoke their mind and then faced a storm of public outrage for it, despite committing no real crime.

Cancel Culture as we know it took shape around 2017, originally with the intention of calling out or curbing behavior deemed inappropriate regarding social justice causes (from combating prejudice to protecting the environment). It really gained traction alongside the rise of the #MeToo movement that year, when survivors of sexual assault and harassment named and shamed their aggressors publicly. In those early instances, "cancellation" was aimed at people who had clearly done wrong – it was a tool of accountability. However, the problem arose when people became lost in the extremely fine line of ethics. What exactly is a crime, and what is not? In the legal world, that might be clearly defined in constitutions and laws. But on the internet, those concepts began to shift and blur.

Like many popular uprisings against perceived "evil" in society, cancel culture brought with it a troubling tendency: the use of entirely emotional arguments without a moment's thought for the consequences. If someone said or did something offensive, the response was immediate public shaming – a virtual mobbing. The offender's entire personhood would be judged by a snapshot of their worst moment. Those few seconds of video or that single regrettable tweet would lead to the notion that everything the person had ever said or done was just as cruel or wrong as that one instance. In the rush to condemn, context, proportion, and forgiveness were lost.

Of course, cancellation doesn't happen only on screens – it has real-life repercussions. But ever since everyone gained a voice on social media, each individual user finds themself in a position of power they never had before. From behind a keyboard, ego grows and courage increases. People say things online they'd never dare say to someone's face. And if they lack courage even for that, no problem: creating an anonymous fake account to sling mud is trivially easy. In this environment, outrage can erupt in an instant, and thousands of voices can join in to dogpile on a target. It feels consequence-free for the participants – a far cry from a face-to-face confrontation.

The main reason I strongly condemn this culture of cancellation is the utter lack of genuine argumentation or dialogue. We're seeing an alarming decline in actual discussion and exchange of ideas. People do not tolerate opinions that diverge from their own. People do not admit the possibility that they might be wrong. And people increasingly confuse facts with opinions, treating any challenge to their viewpoint as a personal attack. This trend is tragic. If there's one thing I learned from Immanuel Kant and try to apply every day, it's the exercise of maturity – which includes the ability to handle disagreement rationally.

It really isn't so hard to make a bit of effort to seek out knowledge and form your own well-founded opinion. That way, when you disagree with someone, you have grounds for it – evidence, logic, a thoughtful perspective – rather than simply condemning them with nothing to back it up. Unfortunately, cancel culture encourages the opposite: knee-jerk condemnation without understanding.

The brevity of thought, the finitude of attention, and frankly the laziness that many exhibit – the unwillingness to contribute anything positive to dialogue – are killing true discourse. And without dialogue, ideas do not evolve. Without the clash of differing thoughts, no one ever progresses. Our ideas should be in constant transformation as we encounter new evidence and perspectives; it's much easier (and more productive) to accept this and learn, rather than to hastily cancel others who are different just because they dare to be authentic when you are not.

Now, let's clarify: none of this is to say that people who truly commit crimes or egregious wrongs don't deserve consequences. It would be madness to equate an online "canceler" (an accuser) with someone who has, say, abused their power or hurt others in real life. If a person commits a crime, the law should handle it. We don't need Twitter mobs – we need common sense and due process. My easing of the burden on some canceled people is not a defense of any and all nonsense that comes out of someone's mouth; it's an affirmation that a person is more than their worst moment. Someone who dares to speak in public – to expose their thoughts to the world – is already a step ahead in courage. We should value that willingness to participate in the discourse, even if we disagree with the content of what they say.

No one should live in fear of making a mistake or expressing an unpopular idea for fear of being cancelled. If that fear rules us, people will simply stop speaking up. They'll hold their true thoughts inside, or only share them in absolute privacy with those they know already agree. And that is dangerous, because it perpetuates prejudice and ignorance. If people only speak to those who already agree with them, bad ideas never get challenged and good ideas never spread. Do you really think ideas are meant to be discussed only with those who already agree with you, or with those who disagree? I'd argue the latter. That is the beauty of democracy and freedom of expression – the clash of viewpoints, out of which truth and progress emerge.

I genuinely hope that in a few decades, this phenomenon of cancel culture will be a memory – that a reader 50 years from now will look back at this chapter's introduction just to recall what "cancel culture" even was, because by then it will have faded away. But right now, it's a force we must reckon with. In a truly liberal society, you are free to do absolutely everything – and that is fantastic. If you commit a crime, you face the law, yes. But short of that, freedom means freedom. No political faction or online mob should get to assign themselves the role of ultimate moral arbiter. (I often notice, for example, how some on the political Left appropriate humanitarian causes as if they exclusively own them – a sheer opportunism that tries to paint opponents as automatically unethical. This isn't limited to one side of the spectrum, either; it's a broader problem in politics today.) We are capable of making our own decisions – we don't need self-appointed commissars telling us who is "good" and who is "evil."

So, is cancellation an attack on democracy? Some argue yes, others no. Rather than give a simple answer, I'd prefer to analyze it. Democracy thrives on the open exchange of ideas; cancel culture thives on shutting ideas down. In that sense, they are at odds. Let's consider a real example to illustrate the dynamic of cancellation and what it does to discourse.

A Personal Example: Conformity Pressure in Youth

One example that stands out in my mind is Brazil's 2018 presidential election. Cancel culture in Brazil hit a peak during that time. Then-candidate (now former President) Jair Bolsonaro had made a number of repugnant public statements – comments widely seen as sexist, homophobic, and racist. Understandably, these statements sparked astronomical reactions. People were angry; I was angry. I was only 15 years old then, and like virtually all my friends, I strongly disagreed with the offensive things Bolsonaro said.

But here's what happened: I felt obligated to vocally oppose absolutely everything associated with him and his political camp. It wasn't enough for me personally to disapprove; I had to show everyone that I was against him. Why? Because among my peers, silence was unacceptable. If I didn't loudly and visibly reject Bolsonaro, I ran the risk of being labeled a "Bolsonarista" (a

Bolsonaro supporter), which was basically a scarlet letter in my social circle. In other words, even though I already disagreed with his views, I felt I had to perform that disagreement to fit in. Do you see how this mirrors cancel culture? The substance mattered less than the performance of alignment with the "correct" position.

This experience taught me a lot about the difference between youth and adulthood in the context of political and social discourse. As a teenager, I believed that every protest, every loud declaration would earn me respect and admiration from my peers. Young people often feel the need to constantly affirm their stances – to prove to their friends, "Hey, I'm on the right side of this issue! I hate what you hate!" Among adults, it's a bit different. No one I know, for instance, seriously agrees with the awful things Bolsonaro said – that's a given. Adults don't need to prove to each other that they find bigotry distasteful; it's assumed. Instead, they're more likely to discuss practicalities – for example, how policy or governance is affected – rather than just vent rage that, in practical terms, changes nothing. Youth, on the other hand, often believe their outspoken protest is the vehicle to change (or at least a ticket to social acceptance). They haven't yet seen how sometimes these virtuous performances can be more about appearing righteous than effecting real change.

I'm not saying this to dismiss young people's passion. Passion is wonderful. I'm saying it as someone who was in that exact position: I felt coerced by social pressure into parroting the "correct" anti-Bolsonaro stance 24/7, into defining myself by what I was against. In fact, I recall calling out or even canceling others with harsh words simply because they didn't speak up against him as fervently as I thought they should. In my mind at that time, it felt like a moral crime for someone to hear the horrible things he said and not become completely enraged. I couldn't fathom a more measured response; nuance felt like complicity to my 15-year-old self.

Now, a few years later, I see how toxic that environment was. It wasn't enough to be privately disgusted by bad behavior; you had to publicly demonstrate outrage or risk being ostracized. This created an atmosphere of fear where people started self-censoring or simply staying silent on everything, unless they were among trusted friends. After all, if even failing to condemn quickly enough could get you labeled and attacked, why risk saying anything at all? This is why I circle back to the concept of freedom I defined earlier: freedom is everything that does not violate another's freedom. Freedom is not "your opinion doesn't align with the prevailing one, so you will be shamed for it." Yet in those moments, that's exactly how society behaved.

Many people, not just teenagers, are now making the decision to stay silent. They hold their tongues, avoid posting, avoid raising a hand – they prefer to lay low rather than become a target. But remember: opinions are not innate; we are not born with them fully formed. We develop our ideas by engaging with the world. If we become too afraid to voice our thoughts, we lose the opportunity to have them challenged and refined. If we don't face the fear of potential backlash, we might never say what we truly think in a public space. And here arises an ENORMOUS problem for the future: What becomes of our democracy if it's no longer a union of different ideas? If only one viewpoint is deemed acceptable and everyone else is shouted down or scared off, how do we make any progress as a society?

Freedom of speech and thought means nothing if people are too afraid to actually exercise it. If you fear confrontation – if the mere thought of someone disagreeing with you or calling you out rattles you to your core – then you might fall permanently silent on all the things that truly matter to you. You pre-emptively cancel yourself. And losing your voice like that is tantamount to losing your very self, your autonomy. You become "annulled" as the spokesperson for your own life, essentially surrendering the driver's seat of your existence.

One of the beautiful aspects of growing up (perhaps the most beautiful) is that you can finally stop trying to please everyone. As teenagers, most of us desperately wanted to fit in – we'd go to parties we hated, drink when we didn't want to, wear clothes we thought were awful – all just to avoid being judged by our peers. Adulthood, ideally, is when you start expressing your genuine feelings, opinions, desires, and beliefs without that crippling fear of rejection. But if you let the specter of cancellation haunt you, if you remain overly affected by the possibility of social backlash, you gradually lose the joy that comes with being your own person. The truth is, no matter what you do, someone will always judge you. You could be a saint and there'd still be a corner of the internet calling you a villain. So if judgment is inevitable, why not endure it for being who you truly are, rather than for a pretend version of yourself?

Let's dig a bit into the psychology behind this fear. Consider the case of a young woman – call her Laura. She once experienced a very public cancellation: hundreds of critical comments flooding her social media, big influencer accounts sharing her alleged "mistake" far and wide. The damage was done – her reputation tarnished, her psyche scarred. Those hateful posts and memes about her are out there forever, a fixed record of public shaming. But here's the question: why can't Laura stop thinking about it even now, long after the internet's attention has moved on? The event was finite – a few days or weeks of infamy – yet she torments herself with it continuously, letting it grow into something psychologically larger than it ever was in reality.

To explain this, we have to acknowledge a basic human instinct: the desire to belong and to be esteemed by our group. As one psychological insight puts it, "The safest thing is always to align oneself with the dominant opinion." In evolutionary terms, standing out from the tribe was dangerous; being cast out of the tribe could be fatal. We carry a deep-seated fear of being isolated or deemed unworthy by our community. What online cancellation does is hijack that primal fear – it attacks a person's social identity and moral standing. The cancel mob isn't just saying "you're wrong"; they're often saying "you're a bad person, and you don't belong with us."

That's why it feels so devastating. It's an attack on one's very morality and membership in the human community.

Compounding the issue is the way people consume information today. In Brazil (as in many places), we aren't a culture of deep readers these days. Many will see a scandalous headline, skim a 280-character tweet, or hear a juicy gossip snippet, and consider that sufficient knowledge to pass judgment. Superficial information spreads like wildfire and solidifies into "truth" in the public mind. Details? Context? Who needs those! For example, I remember an incident where a public figure's quote was taken out of context on a popular Instagram news page; within hours, thousands of comments were calling for that person's head, when in fact the original message was misunderstood. It didn't matter – the mob smelled blood and that was enough. In situations like this, activists online often leap into action before verifying facts, misunderstanding or misrepresenting what was said in the first place.

There are countless such examples of people being misunderstood and unfairly attacked over something trivial or out-of-context. In each of these cases, what happened is that the self-proclaimed activist or moral police took the place of what should have been a more measured, truth-seeking approach. The ethical intellectual – the person who is committed to truth, nuance, and dialogue – gets pushed aside. In comes the reactionary who values virtue-signaling over truth. And when cancellation enters, any remaining chance of genuine debate exits. It's completely compromised. Once the witch hunt begins, there's no discussion, no exchange – just a verdict delivered by the mob.

From a critical standpoint, if one can step back from this surface-level activism and instead commit to seeking truth, something interesting happens: one often becomes happier. I say this from experience. Letting go of the need to control the world's every injustice – to call out every transgression, to react to every offensive remark – can be liberating. You start to understand that the world is not yours to police. That doesn't mean you stop caring about important causes; it means you recognize your limitations and choose your battles with care and personal conviction. By this point in my life, I have a much clearer sense of which causes truly matter to me – the ones I am willing to dedicate my time and energy to – and which causes are better handled by others who are truly passionate about them. This focus has made me more effective and more at peace.

Let me be clear: I'm not advocating for apathy or saying "stop caring about the world." Far from it. I'm saying that your chances of actually making a difference are greater if you aim your efforts in a focused direction. You can't fight every fight; none of us can. But if you pick one (or a few) and pour your soul into it – if you make it your truth – then fight with all you've got. And if it's truly your deeply held truth, you need not fear the backlash. When you know why you're fighting, when you're grounded in principles, then no amount of judgment or rumors or cancellation can derail you. You become somewhat immune to the noise, because you have an internal compass.

Living this way – fighting for what you believe in – leads to living a life you chose, not one dictated by the fleeting approval of others. You stop worrying about whether you meet external expectations, especially the unreasonable ones. A silly example: you won't lose sleep over whether you followed back that famous person who followed you on social media, especially if you don't actually agree with their content. (In the past, I might have felt obligated to follow them out of polite reciprocity or fear of offending, even if their values clashed with mine. Now I couldn't care less – and it's liberating.) You realize that if someone followed you just to get a follow-back, that's their issue, not yours. Likewise, you stop caring if your political or religious views diverge from your friend group's consensus. In high school, that divergence might have caused social suicide; in adult life, it's often precisely where interesting conversation begins. And from genuine, respectful disagreement, cancellation simply doesn't arise. In truth, the most damaging form of "cancellation" isn't the kind that happens on Twitter or in gossip circles – it's the kind that happens in your own mind. It's self-cancellation: the martyrdom complex, the weight of suppressing yourself. Once you free yourself from that, any external controversy seems minor. It almost ceases to exist in any meaningful way, because it doesn't define you or occupy your thoughts beyond a few minutes of annoyance. After all, here's a humbling reality: you are not that important to occupy more than a few minutes of a stranger's thoughts. People move on. The internet moves on insanely fast. The permanence of cancel-culture shaming is overstated – it's our internalization of it that makes it permanent.

I speak from the other side of the tunnel: I only truly became a relieved, confident person once I stopped pretending – pretending to always agree, pretending to care about things I didn't, pretending to be someone I wasn't. Truth – with a capital T – became my aim. Truth in myself (being honest about who I am and what I value), truth in others (seeking to really understand them beyond my prejudices), and truth in circumstances (looking for facts, context, and nuance). This dedication to truth is both a personal ethic and a shield against the temptations of cancel culture.

As a matter of fact, one of my favorite quotes about the modern internet era comes from author Umberto Eco, who famously said something to the effect that the internet has given voice to legions of idiots. In full, he said that social media allows a crowd of imbeciles to speak with the same authority as a Nobel Prize winner – it's the "invasion of the idiots." It sounds harsh, but what he's getting at is the way online platforms amplify uninformed, snap judgments. The web allows anyone to broadcast outrage or police someone else's language without having to do anything constructive or commit to any real-life principles. And sadly, human beings like to judge others. We love it, if we're being honest. There's a certain thrill in it – a moment where the person casting judgment feels pure, elevated, righteous. (I'll note, as a woman, that often women are the harshest judges of other women – we see this play out in cancel culture a lot, where female public figures are torn down by other females over personal choices, appearance, etc. It's painful, but it's pervasive.) That moment of judgment can feel like a sort of transcendence – you project all your insecurities and dark parts onto someone else, condemn them, and by contrast you feel morally spotless. It's an illusion, of course, and a toxic one.

In an environment like this, how do we find a way back to understanding and positivity? Part of the answer lies in broadening our perspective and recognizing our shared humanity, which is something I learned through other aspects of life – like religion, travel, and connecting with others on a deeper level. Let's explore that, because it's directly related to overcoming the kind of negativity that cancel culture feeds on.

Broadening Perspectives: Religion, Travel, and Humility

We humans are, at our core, storytellers. We always have been. Our ancestors sat around fires weaving narratives to explain the world around them. Even today, we construct stories about our lives and our experiences to make sense of them – and when we're depressed or anxious, those stories can become distorted, overly negative, or self-defeating. This storytelling nature is central to both religion and science – two realms often seen in opposition, but which actually have a lot in common in this regard.

Consider religion. Organized religion provided humanity's earliest frameworks for explaining the unexplainable. Thousands of years ago, human life was far more intimately entwined with the whims of nature. Imagine living in a time when a thunderstorm or a drought could feel like a personal wrath from the skies, or a blessing from beyond – when you had no scientific explanation for earthquakes or eclipses. Nature was at once awe-inspiring and terrifying. It fed you with game and crops and water, yet it could destroy your village without warning. To make sense of this duality, early humans did what humans do best: they created symbolic stories. They personified nature into gods and spirits. Water, sun, rain, death – each got a narrative and a deity: Poseidon ruled the seas, Apollo the sun, Zeus the thunder, and so on. By telling these stories, people found a way to relate to the forces controlling their lives. The world became less random and more negotiable – maybe if you pleased the rain god, the rains would come on time.

From the very beginning, then, myth and religion were about answering the big mysteries that no one – not even now – has fully solved. Where do we come from? Why do the sun and moon dance across the sky? Why do we feel pain and joy? What happens after we die? These are questions that, in one form or another, every culture has asked. And before the age of modern science, mythology, philosophy, and religion were the main tools to grapple with them. One of the great errors we can make today is to look back at those ancient stories and scoff. It's easy, from the vantage of our technology-saturated 21st century lives, to dismiss, say, the Greek pantheon or indigenous creation tales as "silly" or "naive." But that's incredibly narrow-minded – it's judging a different culture's worldview only by the standards of our own. We all do this to some extent (it's a human habit), but it's something we should catch and correct in ourselves. Every culture's stories made sense in context. They were doing the best they could with the information they had. And in a poetic sense, they often contain emotional or metaphorical truths that resonate even now.

As time went on, religion took on new roles. It was no longer just about explaining thunder and harvests; it became a way to organize society, to establish power dynamics and social orders. Kings and emperors ruled by divine right. Churches and mosques laid down rules for how communities should live, sometimes oppressively so. In the modern era, we see how religion (or any rigid ideology, really) can be used to control and even imprison minds. Any system of belief that has very fixed ideals and dogmas can end up infringing on personal freedom – even if it began as a voluntary association. Ironically, this can make religion in practice similar to the most zealous social movements: any structure that demands absolute adherence to an ideology can become stifling. (Cancel culture has its dogmas too, if you think about it – certain words you can't say, complex issues reduced to moral binaries, etc.) Now, I'm not attacking faith itself – being part of a faith or not is a personal choice, and many find meaning and community there. I'm saying that the power structures and extreme orthodoxies can be problematic when they suppress individual thought and liberty.

On the flip side, despite their differences, religion and science share a surprising common ground: both are fueled by an immense fascination with the unknown. The devoutly religious gaze at nature or the stars and feel wonder about the Creator's design; scientists gaze at the same and feel wonder about the laws governing it. Both are asking the big question: Who or what made all this? How does it work? Why are we here? It's no surprise that both religion and science evoke such awe – they are each grappling, in their own way, with the infinite. And it is daunting work for either the priest or the physicist to pin down answers about a universe that is so much larger and stranger than us. In that sense, a monk and a biologist have something profound in common: humility in the face of a mystery.

This brings me to a more personal level: how do we as individuals keep perspective and resist the pull of negativity or harsh judgment? One answer for me has been stepping outside of my own bubble – literally leaving my home environment, traveling, and seeing how other people live. Travel is a remarkable antidote to arrogance and narrow-mindedness. It makes you humble. When you travel, you're confronted with how vast the world really is and how many ways there are to live a life. You see that your way of thinking is just one of countless ways, and that many people who think differently from you are not evil or stupid – they're just coming from a different context.

I used to think, for example, that my culture or my way had figured out the best approach to life's problems. But when you travel, you realize that at the end of the day, we're all the same in the broad strokes. Every single person on this planet is going through some version of the same handful of experiences and emotions. We all seek happiness; we all try to avoid suffering. Some chase fulfillment through hard work and career achievements. Others, overwhelmed by pain, escape into drugs or alcohol. Some find purpose in family, others in art, others sadly lose their way and even consider ending their lives. On the more extreme edges, at any given moment, there are people fighting for one more day in a hospital bed while others waste a day scrolling on their phones feeling miserable for no apparent reason.

Travel throws all these contrasts into sharp relief. You might meet someone from a remote village who has none of your material luxuries yet radiates contentment – and it makes you question where your discontent comes from. You might encounter cultures where community and family are prioritized above all, and realize how lonely individualism can be. You might see great poverty and realize how much you actually have to be grateful for. All of this gives you perspective. It becomes harder to sit in judgment of others when you've seen how circumstances shape people. It becomes harder to indulge in the negative thought that "my life is uniquely awful" when you've seen real suffering and also real joy in places you never expected.

To tie it back, broad perspectives help inoculate us against the knee-jerk negativity of phenomena like cancel culture. When you realize how big the world is, you understand that your view (or your group's view) is not the only one – and that's okay. You become less inclined to demonize someone for thinking differently. You also become less likely to wallow in your own negativity because you see that life has ups and downs for everyone, everywhere.

There's a quote by the psychologist Jordan B. Peterson that I find relevant here, from a talk he gave in 2017 about free speech and truth. He said:

"Life is suffering. Love is the desire to see unnecessary suffering ameliorated. Truth is the handmaiden of love. Dialogue is the pathway to truth. Humility is recognition of personal insufficiency and the willingness to learn. To learn is to die voluntarily and be born again, in great ways and small. Speech must be untrammeled so that dialogue can take place; so that we can all humbly learn, so that truth can serve love, so that suffering can be ameliorated; so that we can all stumble forward toward the kingdom of God."

I know that's a mouthful, but look at how beautifully he connects these concepts: suffering, love, truth, dialogue, humility. In essence, he's saying: Yes, life has pain. Love motivates us to reduce each other's pain. To truly do that, we need truth, and to find truth we need dialogue – open, free dialogue. That requires humility – acknowledging we don't have all the answers and being willing to listen and learn. And for dialogue to happen, speech must be free. We have to allow people to talk, even if they sometimes say stupid or wrong things, because that's the only way we all improve and alleviate the unnecessary suffering in the world. Cancel culture, for all the good intentions some of its proponents might have, utterly undermines this process. It trades humility for smugness, dialogue for diatribe, truth for moral grandstanding. We can do better than that – and it starts by broadening our horizons, checking our egos, and remembering the fundamental love for humanity that should underlie our actions.

Having explored how cancel culture fosters negativity by shrinking our world view, let's turn to another facet of negativity: the kind that brews in our personal lives when we become isolated or when we don't take care of our mental well-being. If broad perspective and free dialogue are antidotes to societal negativity, stability and connection are antidotes to personal negativity.

The Quiet Power of Social Connection

Through my own struggles, I've come to believe that the path to recovering from depression – and, more importantly, the path to sustaining mental health – is not about chasing some constant euphoric happiness. It's about finding stability and contentment in the everyday. When I talk about keeping "mental health in check," I mean attaining a life that feels normal (in a good way). Not every day is bliss, not everything is perfect – but overall, there's balance.

The first steps toward that balanced life are almost deceptively simple: being at peace with yourself and tending to your basic physical needs. We often talk about mental health and physical health like they're separate, but they're deeply intertwined. In my view, there are three essential pillars for well-being: sleep, nutrition, and physical activity. These three have been discussed to death by everyone from doctors to Instagram influencers, and I myself have harped on them on social media for years – because they matter. And of those three, the one we tend to neglect most is sleep. It sounds trite, but so many problems in life feel insurmountable when you're sleep-deprived and miraculously become manageable after a good night's rest. If you find yourself asking, "Why do I feel so off? Why is everything collapsing?" sometimes the answer is as straightforward as: you haven't been getting enough quality sleep. Sleep affects mood, concentration, appetite, energy – everything. It is profound and yet we often treat it as a luxury or an afterthought.

Now, it's worth noting that in recent times an interesting paradox has emerged: even as we acknowledge those pillars of health, society has developed a kind of obsession with "perfect" health routines. You see it in endless YouTube morning routine videos, or the Instagram trend of the "That Girl" aesthetic (you know, the girl who wakes up at 5am, drinks a green smoothie, journals, runs 5 miles, meditates, has flawless skin, etc.). While having healthy habits is great, this pressure to be the epitome of wellness can actually create anxiety and a sense of inadequacy. It's as if we've turned self-care into another competition or performance. The whole point of a healthy routine is to support your life, not to become your life. There's a subtle but important difference: one path glorifies a kind of perfectionism, the other appreciates the beauty of a quiet, steady life. A life that may not look glamorous on camera, but is rich and fulfilling because it has balance.

I speak from experience, because I've swung on that pendulum. I've lived the disciplined life of rigid routines and lofty goals, pushing myself relentlessly. And I've also experienced times where I let go and embraced simpler, quieter living. The big revelation for me was that obsession – even with something as positive as health or success – is still obsession. It can become destructive if it causes you to neglect other core aspects of being human. And one of those aspects, which I learned the hard way not to overlook, is social connection.

We are inherently social creatures – we need other people (even we introverts need close friends or family, just in manageable doses!). I have dedicated an entire chapter elsewhere in my work to social relationships because I cannot overstate how essential it is to cultivate meaningful bonds with others. Let me illustrate this with a personal story:

When I moved from my home in Goiânia (a city in Brazil) to New York City, I thought I had everything I needed within myself. I carried with me all my ambition, independence, and determination – qualities that had defined me and brought me success up to that point. I was (and am) very career-driven and focused. Those traits helped me get into Columbia University and survive the intense academic pressure there. I prided myself on being relentless in pursuit of my dreams. However, once I landed in New York, I realized something that shook me: my ability to thrive all those years wasn't due to ambition alone. It was largely due to the environment that nurtured me. Back in Goiânia, I had the constant presence of friends and family. Weekend gatherings, casual hangouts, the proverbial shoulder to lean on – these were all around me, effortlessly and abundantly. I had a safety net of belonging. It was so woven into my everyday life that I never even recognized it as a factor in my success or happiness. It was like air – invisible yet vital.

New York, in contrast, was a different universe. I might as well have moved to a different planet. Suddenly, I found myself in the so-called "capital of the world", but with no familiar faces, no familiar customs, no native language jokes or cultural shorthand. I was a small fish not just in a big pond, but in an ocean. I thought my ambition and grit would carry me through anything, but day to day, something intangible was holding me back: I was lonely. I was unmoored. The deep, close, long-standing connections I had always taken for granted were now 5,000 miles away, living their lives in another hemisphere. I especially felt this void when winter came. (Having grown up in Brazil, I wasn't prepared for how brutal and isolating a Northeast winter can be.) When the cold descended, life in New York changed. It wasn't just the temperature; it was like the whole world became more distant. People hurry from one building to another to avoid the chill; the streets empty out except for determined commuters. Walking outside – which used to be something I loved, a way to enjoy the city – turned into a misery of shivering and dodging icy wind. If you grow up in that climate, perhaps you build an inner resilience and, importantly, you have a lifetime of memories making the cold fun or meaningful (like childhood snow days, holiday gatherings by a warm fireplace, etc.). You also typically have a support system: family who will drive you or pick you up if you're stuck in a blizzard, a warm home stocked with blankets and cocoa, friends you've known since kindergarten to come over and watch movies. In my case, I had none of that in New York. My family was not there. I lived in a student apartment with basic heating (which sometimes failed). I didn't have the right winter gear initially, and I certainly didn't have a car or a long-time friend who could rescue me if I got stuck somewhere in a snowstorm. My support system was an ocean away, and a phone call, though nice, isn't the same as a hug or a hot meal with people who love you.

Those winters in New York were, to put it bluntly, incredibly lonely. The worst periods of my life. It's not that I didn't know anyone at all – I had classmates, and I made some friends – but these were new relationships, still budding, not the kind of friends who feel like family. Meanwhile, my actual lifelong friends and family members were waking up under a tropical sun, going about life as usual. I'd scroll through social media seeing them at a barbecue or a birthday party back home, and I'd be sitting alone in a tiny dorm room watching the early sunset at 4 PM, hearing the wind howl outside. It felt like the world was moving on without me, joyously, while I was stuck in a cold, dark limbo.

What this isolation taught me – in the most visceral way – is that friendships and social connections can be more important than anything else, including ambition and willpower. I had never struggled with motivation before; I was always full of plans and drive. But in that lonely environment, I often found myself unmotivated, even lethargic. It puzzled me at first. Why can't I just push through like I always used to? The answer was that the human element was missing. I was like a plant trying to grow without sunlight.

Psychologically, we outsource a lot of our sanity and motivation to our social environment – more than we realize. There's a concept I encountered (during one of those late-night deep dives into psychology literature, prompted by my own state of mind) that people remain mentally healthy not merely because of the solidity of their own mind, but because those around them constantly remind them how to think, act, and even feel in sane ways. In a community, if you start veering off into strange behavior or negative patterns, others (even without knowing they're doing it) will nudge you back: a friend might say "Hey, you haven't been out in a while, let's go for a walk" when you're getting too depressed, or a coworker might give you a puzzled look if you start ranting incoherently, which cues you that maybe you need to check yourself. These are subtle feedback loops that keep us grounded. In psychological terms, we "outsource the problem of sanity" to our network of peers.

Think about how we learn as children: if a kid does something socially inappropriate, ten adults and older kids immediately correct them – "Don't do that, it's not nice," or "That's not how we behave." Bit by bit, that child's wild psyche is shaped into something that can function among others. We often forget that this shaping process never really stops. As adults, we still get shaped – just more subtly. The consensus of our friends, our colleagues, our community at large – it all acts as a guiding force. We don't have to be perfectly self-sufficient islands of rationality; we get by with a little help (or a lot of help) from our friends, as the song goes.

When I became socially isolated, I lost those balancing forces. There was no one to notice if I was sleeping too much (a sign of brewing depression) or too little. No familiar face to say "how's it going?" and pull me out of my spiraling thoughts. Sure, I could call someone, but I often didn't, because I didn't want to worry them or admit I was struggling. It's ironic: I was in a city of 8 million people, yet I felt more isolated than ever.

I started noticing something fascinating when I did manage to socialize: even a couple of hours of genuine conversation with someone could lift a huge weight off my mind. If I voiced my worries or problems out loud to a friend, many times I'd find that by the end of the chat, those problems seemed smaller or more manageable. Sometimes the friend offered advice or comfort, but sometimes all they did was listen – yet in speaking, I had sort of organized my own thoughts and emotions better. I later came across a line that resonated: "We mostly think by talking." In other words, we need to talk to others to process our experiences. It helps us remember what's important and let go of what's not. It helps us hear ourselves and realize when we're being irrational. It's one reason therapy works (therapy is a structured form of talking and being heard), but it's also why having a trusted friend or family member to confide in is priceless.

I even observed this phenomenon in others around me. There was a classmate of mine who, in the first semester, rarely spoke to anyone and seemed stuck in a very negative mindset – always complaining in his journal or looking gloomy. Over time, another student group kind of adopted him; they'd invite him out for coffee, include him in study sessions. As he slowly engaged more socially, I noticed he spent less time voicing negative thoughts and more time actually working on solutions or talking about neutral/positive topics. It was like night and day. By being more social, he unconsciously shifted from ruminating on problems to problem-solving and moving forward. In another instance, I had a friend who was going through a lot – personal loss, academic stress, health issues – and she tended to retreat and isolate when overwhelmed. I made a point to visit her dorm room regularly and just chat, or drag her out for a quick lunch. At first, she would only vent about negative things (which was completely understandable given what she was facing). I let her pour it out. But I also gently steered conversations towards some of the good things still in her life – her talents, funny memories, small wins. Over a few months, the balance of what she talked about shifted. She started bringing up positive observations on her own. She hadn't magically solved all her issues, but by reconnecting socially, she got back in tune with parts of life that were not miserable. She later told me that those conversations were a lifeline, not because I gave any particularly brilliant advice, but because through talking she "felt normal again."

All of this reinforced a deep conviction in me: staying connected with our fellow humans is critical for our brain to perceive life more positively. Isolation breeds a kind of tunnel vision where your problems echo back louder and louder in your own head. Connection shines light into that tunnel, revealing that the world is bigger – that you are bigger – than just your worries. In a community, even a community of two, burdens feel lighter. This doesn't mean every introvert needs a million friends; it means we all need meaningful connections in whatever dosage is right for us. We need people who remind us of reality when our minds distort things, who challenge us, who support us, who laugh with us (laughter especially – nothing flips a bad day around like a good laugh with a friend).

It's fascinating – and a bit sobering – how our minds and sanity are to some extent a social construct. One psychiatrist I read noted that if someone is behaving in a somewhat eccentric or even neurotic way, as long as they have a social circle that tolerates them, they can get by in society because that circle will keep them in check (like, "Oh that's just Bob, he hates crowds, we'll invite him in a way he's comfortable," etc.). But if that person loses their social network, their quirks can escalate into serious dysfunction because there's no feedback mechanism. It made me realize that even our identity is forged in relation to others. We're not separate islands; we're more like points in an endless web, each held in place by strings connecting to others. Cut the strings, and you start to drift.

So, on the societal level, we talked about how negativity and judgment (like cancel culture) can tear us apart. On the personal level, I want to highlight how connection and communication are the opposite of that – they pull us together and help heal or stave off the internal negativity that can manifest as anxiety, depression, or despair. If cancel culture is society's impulse to expel, good social bonds are the antidote that embraces. They say, "You're not alone, you belong, and together we'll get through this."

Now, even with supportive relationships and a healthy lifestyle, many of us still struggle with negativity in the form of internal narratives and habits that keep us stuck. In the final part of this chapter, I want to talk about those patterns – how we sometimes almost force ourselves to stay sad or stuck – and how we can take steps to let the brain and body do what they naturally want to do: heal.

CHAPTER 8

The Brain Will Heal If You Let It

Overcoming Self-Imposed Negativity

I have a mantra of sorts: the brain will heal if you let it. What I mean is that our minds and bodies have remarkable self-healing capabilities – but we often stand in their way. Sometimes we do so out of ignorance, sometimes out of fear, sometimes because we've unknowingly become comfortable in our discomfort.

I'll start with a metaphor. In religious lore, there's the story of the Israelites who escaped slavery in Egypt and journeyed to the Promised Land. But to get there, they had to wander for 40 years in the desert. I once heard someone compare personal growth to that journey, saying, "You don't get to the Promised Land by Uber." There is no quick, cushy ride to lasting happiness or fulfilment. Happiness isn't a pill you can swallow (no matter how much we wish it were), and it's not as simple as doing one 30-day yoga challenge or reading one self-help book. It requires going through the desert – facing discomfort, uncertainty, and hardship.

In my own quest for better mental health, I've had to traverse many little "deserts." A desert can be a sleepless night you tough out because you're trying to wean yourself off the sleeping pills you've relied on. A desert can be a weekend of digital detox, enduring the itch to check your phone every five minutes and sitting with your thoughts instead. Training for a marathon was one of my deserts – those early morning runs in the freezing New York cold, each step a battle between the part of me that wanted to quit and the part that urged me on. Or when I decided to simplify my diet to break some unhealthy food habits – eating very plain, healthy meals day in and day out felt like a desert of blandness at first, as my brain craved the excitement of sugar or junk food.

Why do I call these things deserts? Because they are uncomfortable. They force you out of the cozy, familiar confines of habit and vice. They test you. But on the other side of a desert is something beautiful:

growth. When you come out of that sleepless night without your usual pill, you realize, "Hey, I actually survived, maybe I can do it again." After a digital detox, you might discover you love painting or writing or walking when your brain isn't constantly fed dopamine from a screen. After enduring miles of training, you hit the finish line of a race and that victory is real – infinitely more satisfying than any fleeting comfort you gave up. The finish line (the "Promised Land") is Instagrammable – you stand there with your medal or your newfound peace or your healthy body, and it looks like a triumph. But the marathon to get there – that long conversation between you and your desire to give up – that's where the real work and transformation happen. From mile 35 onwards (metaphorically speaking), you're basically negotiating with your own soul about whether you can handle being happy. Because yes, happiness takes handling – it demands strength.

Modern conversations about mental health have thankfully moved beyond just the absence of mental illness. Today we recognize that mental health is tied to wellbeing and quality of life, not just "not being depressed" or "not having anxiety." It's about a kind of internal equilibrium. When psychologists define mental health now, they talk about the ability to develop your skills and interests, to cope with normal stresses, to work productively, and to contribute to your community. It's about having a sense of purpose and maintaining fulfilling relationships. It's about being able to experience the full range of emotions – yes, even the negative ones – and navigate them without getting stuck.

In other words, mental health is about resilience and balance. It's having your own tools to take care of yourself and to coexist with your environment (friends, family, coworkers, society) in a positive way. It doesn't mean you're happy all the time – that's impossible. It means when you have a bad day or a sorrow or a conflict, you have ways to process it, people to talk to, habits that help you recover. It means you're not a leaf blown about by every wind of emotion; you have roots to steady you.

One big obstacle to achieving this balance is that we often ignore our mental well-being until it's in crisis. We're pretty good at reacting to physical pain – if you twist your ankle badly, you'll probably ice it or see a doctor, not just walk on it for weeks. But when it comes to our mind, we have a tendency to brush off early warning signs. If you start feeling unusually down for days, if you're persistently anxious, if you can't sleep night after night, if you find yourself withdrawing from friends or lashing out in anger – these are all like mental sprains and fractures. And yet many people will say, "Ah, it's just stress" or "I'm just in a funk, it'll pass," and they keep limping along on that injured psyche without seeking help or making changes. We downplay psychological pain in a way we never would physical pain, partly because of stigma and partly because a broken mind is harder to see than a broken arm.

In my practice (and personal life), I see every day how the body and mind are one. Chronic physical issues like hormonal imbalances, vitamin deficiencies, or even gut problems can deeply affect your mood and thoughts. Conversely, mental struggles like anxiety and depression can manifest physically – fatigue, headaches, weakened immune system, you name it. There's research showing that over time, mental disorders like depression can even make one more susceptible to illnesses, and vice versa. So when we talk about "health," it has to be holistic. Mental health surrounds and permeates all aspects of life; it's like a cloud (or aura, if you will) around everything we do and experience.

That means everyone should care about mental health – not just those diagnosed with something. You shouldn't wait until you're in a full breakdown to pay attention to your psychological well-being, just as you shouldn't wait for a heart attack to start caring about your heart. Think of it as maintenance. We all want to be well enough to play our roles in daily life – whether that role is student, parent, worker, friend, or anything else – and to enjoy life's pleasures.

A crucial part of mental wellness is accepting that uncomfortable emotions are part of real life. No one is happy all the time, and that's okay. Feelings like sadness, anger, fear, boredom – they are signals. They're telling us something, and often they're transient if we acknowledge them. The problem comes when we encounter these uncomfortable feelings and we panic, thinking, "Oh no, I must not feel this, make it go away now." In a frantic bid to escape emotional pain, many people turn to what I call numbing behaviors: drinking alcohol, using drugs, overeating comfort food, endlessly scrolling on the phone, or even misusing prescription meds. In the short term, these might provide relief or distraction. But in the long run, they all carry costs – health issues, addiction, deeper social isolation, and a worsened ability to cope. Essentially, by trying to numb ourselves, we often harm ourselves, and by doing so we also hurt our relationships with others (someone who's drunk or zoned out all the time isn't exactly nurturing their friendships or responsibilities).

The first step out of that trap is acceptance: recognizing that real life comes with good and bad feelings, and that these feelings ebb and flow like the seasons or a Ferris wheel. You won't always be up, but neither will you always be down. And crucially, feelings are not facts, nor are they destiny. They're experiences. If you feel sad, it doesn't mean your life is objectively sad or that you'll be sad forever; it means in this moment, sadness is in you – and like any visitor, it can be understood and it will eventually depart. When you accept this, you can start to approach your emotions more curiously and less judgmentally: "Okay, I'm really anxious today, what might be triggering it? What can I do to support myself through it?" This mindset turns you into an observer and caretaker of your own mind, rather than a helpless victim of it.

Once you're observing your feelings, you can develop strategies to deal with them. This might mean learning relaxation techniques for anxiety, or scheduling social activities when you notice you're isolating too much, or using creativity or exercise as an outlet for frustration. There's no one-size-fits-all answer – it's a personal toolkit you build over time. Some people journal to process emotions, others pray or meditate, others need a good workout to reset their brain chemistry. But the key is not letting emotions dominate you; you work with them, listen to them, but you don't hand them the steering wheel to your life.

I'm a big believer that the future of mental health – and really the present, starting now – is in prevention and early intervention. It's much easier to take small steps to maintain your mental equilibrium than to pick up the pieces after a total collapse. In practical terms, this means paying attention to those subtle warning signs I mentioned. If you notice you're in a persistently bad mood, chronically irritable, always tired despite rest, not sleeping well, avoiding social interaction, or maybe eating way too much or having no appetite – take that seriously. These might or might not be full-blown disorder symptoms, but either way they're waving a yellow flag that says "hey, something's off with your lifestyle or environment or internal state, address it." Don't just push through month after month and let it become your new normal. Life is too short to live in unnecessary pain or under a grey cloud that might be lifted with some changes.

It's striking how many mental health issues are connected to how we live and the world around us. Our environment and lifestyle play a huge role in conditions like anxiety and depression. For instance, if you live in constant stress – maybe a toxic home or a high-pressure job – that's like a plant in poor soil; it's hard to thrive. Or if you never get sunlight or exercise, of course your mind struggles too. On a large scale, we see this in statistics: my country, Brazil, unfortunately has one of the highest rates of depression in the world – the highest in Latin America and second highest in the Americas (after the U.S.) Why? It's not because Brazilians are born predisposed to sadness. It's because of a confluence of socio-economic issues, cultural factors, lifestyle changes, etc. – in short, environment.

Now, none of us can singlehandedly change the broader environment or magically remove all sources of stress from society. What we can do is choose how we respond and structure our own lives within whatever reality we're in. It comes down to choices: how do I reconcile my personal desires with the demands of the world around me? Where do I rank myself on my list of priorities (hint: if you're always last, that's a problem)? How much do I respect my own limits and well-being when making decisions? These are deeply personal questions, but they determine whether we are active participants in our mental health or passive passengers.

Let me address a modern factor that weighs particularly on younger generations: social media. We touched on cancel culture, which largely plays out on social media, but there's another aspect: the endless comparison and body image issues. Study after study has shown that heavy social media use is linked to higher rates of body dissatisfaction, especially among girls and young women. It's not hard to see why – your feed is full of filtered, curated images of seemingly perfect people. Even if you know intellectually that it's curated, emotionally you start feeling inadequate. For some, this spirals into compulsive behaviors or eating disorders like anorexia or bulimia. The constant bombardment of "ideal" bodies and lives can make anyone start to question their own worth or looks. So when we talk about environment and lifestyle factors, we have to include our digital environment too. If scrolling Instagram is making you hate your body or life, be mindful of that. Curate your feed or take breaks. Your brain wasn't evolved to handle the social comparison of seeing the highlight reel of 1000 people's lives every day.

Another point I want to emphasize: as wonderful as medical science is, pills alone won't fix a broken life. Antidepressants, anti-anxiety meds, etc., can be lifesaving tools – they can give you a window of relief, a platform on which to start rebuilding your habits and thoughts. I have taken medication at points, and I'm grateful it exists. But I'm under no illusion that medication can carry me to the finish line by itself. It's more like a painkiller for the mind – it dulls the ache, which is important, but it doesn't heal the wound. The healing comes from changes in how you live and think. If someone is in severe depression, yes, medication might be necessary to even get them out of bed. But once they're out of bed, the real work begins: therapy, reconnecting with loved ones, exercising even when it's the last thing they want to do, finding a purpose to get up for, tweaking their diet, maybe quitting that job that's killing them inside, etc. These are the things that address the root causes, which often lie in lifestyle, unresolved trauma, or unhealthy environments.

When I say "the brain will heal if you let it do its job," a lot of that letting comes from establishing a life that supports healing. For me, one of the simplest yet most powerful such supports is routine. Our bodies and brains thrive on a bit of predictability. I know that sounds boring – especially to younger me, who loved spontaneity – but it's true. When you have some structure in your day, your system doesn't have to be on high alert all the time. If you generally sleep, eat, work, and relax around regular times, your body knows what to expect and can regulate itself better. Without any routine, everything feels chaotic – you might overproduce stress hormones because, say, you're pulling all-nighters then crashing randomly. Over time that wears you down. Routine also gives a psychological benefit: a sense of control. Even a small routine, like making your bed in the morning or taking a short walk every afternoon, can anchor you. When life around you feels crazy, those little anchor points remind you that you are in charge of you. They build confidence. And confidence is the enemy of certain kinds of anxiety and despair.

Now, I'm not advocating for a rigid schedule that never changes – that can become its own source of stress. I'm saying a flexible, supportive routine is helpful. And if you're trying to turn your mental health around, don't attempt to do 100 new healthy habits at once. That's a recipe for failure and self-blame. It's much better to prioritize and start somewhere doable. Maybe this month you focus on getting

7-8 hours of sleep consistently. Next month you add a little exercise to your week. Then you work on reducing screen time before bed. Step by step, at your own pace, you build these pillars. Each one gives you some strength and momentum for the next. There's no rush; it's not a competition. Slow progress is still progress.

Everything I've described – the routines, the lifestyle changes, the facing of uncomfortable feelings – are ways of letting your natural healing processes take place. Your brain wants to balance itself. Think about it: if you get a cut on your skin, you don't have to tell it to heal; your body will start clotting the blood, sending white blood cells, knitting the skin back together. Your job is mostly to keep the wound clean and protected so it can do its thing. Similarly, if you're emotionally wounded or mentally overtaxed, your job is to create conditions for healing: maybe that's taking a break, maybe it's talking to a friend, maybe it's consulting a therapist who can guide that healing. If you constantly poke at a wound, it won't heal. Likewise, if you constantly engage in negative behaviors or self-sabotaging thoughts, you don't give your mind the space to recover.

I've observed that many of us – and I was guilty of this – play the victim in our own lives without realizing it. It's like we choose to stay in a place of hardship even when a door to exit is right there. We get so used to complaining and seeing everything in a negative light that even when solutions appear, we unconsciously shy away from them, because solving the problem would mean losing the comfort of that familiar pain or the attention we get from others for being pitiful. It's a harsh thing to admit, but I've seen it enough times, including in myself at times, to know it's real.

Let me share a somewhat silly but illustrative anecdote. A few years ago, I had an acquaintance – let's call her Barbara (a fictitious name) – who was absolutely livid one day because she missed the final theater showing of a film starring her favorite actor. It was one of those limited release situations, one night only. She was ranting and furious: "Life is so unfair! I've waited so long for this and now I missed it! I'll never get another chance to see it on the big screen!" Her anger was almost operatic; you could see it in her face, hear it in her voice.

Being a problem-solver, I stepped in and said, "Hey, maybe all is not lost. Let's see if any theater anywhere near here is still showing it." I went online, checked around, and lo and behold, a cinema in a city about 5 hours' drive away still had a showing later that week. I told Barbara the good news. Now, a 5-hour drive is a lot, but I was in the mood for a spontaneous road trip and frankly happy to help her out. So I said, "If you really want to see it, I'll go with you. We can drive over, make a fun trip of it. And if money's a problem, I'll cover the tickets – consider it an adventure."

For a moment, she was overjoyed and surprised: "Really? You'd do that?" I smiled, "Sure, why not?" So it looked like the problem was solved – easy peasy. But then, almost immediately, she hesitated: "Umm, I don't know… I have a weird feeling about it. Like… I feel like I'm gonna be in danger if I go."

Now, there was no logical basis for this feeling. This was a daytime showing in a decent city we were both somewhat familiar with, and she'd have me with her the whole time. No danger beyond the usual risks of a road trip (and we could manage those). I tried to gently ask what she meant, but she stayed vague: "I can't explain it. I just have a bad feeling. You wouldn't understand." Then she started saying things like, "I know you think I'm making excuses." It became clear that Barbara was looking for reasons not to go – after I had just eliminated the obvious obstacles (lack of time, lack of transport, cost). This incident might seem trivial – it's just a movie, after all – but I found it revealing. Barbara went from a state of extreme negativity and complaint, to having a clear path out of her problem, and she rejected the solution. Why? Because, I suspect, what she really wanted was not to see the movie, but to vent her frustration and maybe get sympathy for it. Solving the problem would rob her of the emotional drama of being wronged by the universe. In her mind, the narrative "I missed it and life sucks" was already set, and weirdly, she was attached to that narrative more than she was to actually fixing it and moving on.

This kind of behavior is more common than we think. People will come up with very reasonable-sounding explanations for why they can't do something that would actually help them, until those explanations run out, and then they resort to the unreasonable or mystical ones ("I have a weird gut feeling" or "I think it's a sign I shouldn't go"). Anything to avoid taking the leap that would resolve their complaint.

I've encountered this pattern in more serious contexts, too. For instance, I had a friend who struggled with an intense fear of water. She couldn't swim and was terrified of even trying. Living in a coastal city, this fear limited a lot of her social activities (no beach trips, no pool parties, always worrying about situations involving water). She frequently lamented this fear, saying she wished she could enjoy the ocean like everyone else. So, trying to help, I offered so many alternatives: we could go to a very shallow pool and just sit in the water to get used to it; we could take a low-pressure adult swim class with supportive instructors; we could even just go to the beach and only let the waves touch our feet to start. Each time, she had a reason to say no. Finally, she told me something that left me speechless: she said she believed her fear was essentially not her fault at all – she blamed it on structural racism. Her reasoning was that because African slaves (ancestors of many Black Brazilians like herself) were historically not allowed leisure or access to learning things like swimming, swimming never became part of Black culture; therefore, she felt no obligation to break that pattern. In her view, her fear was almost an inherited, collective condition – not an individual challenge she could choose to overcome.

Now, I am 100% sensitive to the lasting impacts of historical injustices, and it's true that inequalities can have ripple effects on communities (access to pools, swimming lessons, etc.). But at the end of the day, in today's world, nothing was literally stopping my friend from learning to swim except her own fear and decision. Plenty of Black people do swim. It wasn't a lack of opportunity in the present; it was her mindset. I even gently suggested that maybe talking to a therapist about the fear could help – because it seemed like more than just a social issue, it was a phobia that perhaps had personal roots. She brushed that off too. The possibility of taking responsibility for overcoming her fear was too much; it was safer for her to externalize it as something beyond her control.

This might sound extreme, but think about other scenarios: How many people do you know who insist that their weight is entirely due to genetics or society ("all the women in my family are heavy, I can't help it" or "media pressure makes me overeat")? And yet, they haven't ever earnestly tried sustained moderate exercise and a balanced diet, or if they did, they gave up quickly. Because trying and failing is scary – it's much "easier" to say "It's not in my control. I'm a victim of circumstance."

Or consider the phenomenon of someone who seems to like being sick because it provides an excuse to avoid responsibilities. I knew someone (fortunately not too close to me) who would almost brag about their ailments, because it got them sympathy and let them bow out of everything – work, family events, you name it. If they started to get healthier, I suspect they'd feel a bit lost, because then they'd have to actually face life without that shield of illness. It's a twisted comfort zone, but it is a comfort zone for some.

Earlier in the book I wrote about overprotected children – kids whose parents do everything to shield them from failure or pain. When such kids grow up, they often haven't developed the coping skills for adversity, because they never had to practice them. They can become the kinds of adults who look for others to blame or save them whenever something goes wrong. It's like they internalize, "I can't handle this on my own; someone fix it for me." It's another way we inadvertently force ourselves into helplessness and negativity.

Breaking out of these patterns requires a brutal honesty with oneself. I had to do it too. I had to ask: Am I really doing everything I can to get better? Or am I secretly holding onto my pain because it's easier than stepping into the unknown of improvement? At one point in my depression, I realized I was almost comfortable in my misery – it was a known space, whereas trying to be well was unfamiliar and scary. That was a chilling realization, because it meant the call was coming from inside the house, so to speak. The enemy wasn't just out there (in society or brain chemistry or whatever); part of it was me. My attitudes, my avoidance, my excuses – I was feeding the dark wolf instead of the light one.

So I started changing my narrative. I began telling myself the truth I already knew deep down: that I did have power to improve my situation, that diet and exercise (though hard to start) would eventually make me feel better, that apologizing to someone I'd hurt or forgiving someone who hurt me would lift huge weights off my chest, that engaging with a therapist or even certain books could give me tools to cope. I had to stop avoiding the very truths and tasks that I knew would lead to a lighter life.

Yes, sometimes it meant swallowing my pride (like admitting I needed help), sometimes it meant swallowing discomfort (like dragging myself to the gym or forcing myself to socialize when I wanted to hide). It was far from instant happiness – it was slow and incremental. But each small step proved to me that my victim narrative was false. I wasn't completely powerless. Maybe life dealt me certain cards (maybe you have a predisposition to depression, or you grew up poor, or you face discrimination – those are real disadvantages). But within my sphere, there were choices I could make to better my odds.

Arguing without logic – which I used to do when I was defensive – got me nowhere. Complaining got me sympathy but no solutions. Blaming society or others might have often had truth in it, but it didn't change my reality day to day. At some point, I had to decide: do I want to be angry, or do I want to be better? Do I want to be "right," or do I want to be well? Because you can shout about how unfair everything is and you might be right – but you might also be miserable. Sometimes, to get better, you have to let go of the righteousness of your complaint and focus on what you can do.

And let me tell you, when you start owning your life in this way, it's incredibly empowering. It's also humbling, because you can't blame anyone else if things don't improve – you have to face yourself. But that humility is part of maturity. It's the "exercise of maturity" I mentioned earlier, applied inwardly.

I won't lie: choosing responsibility is often painful at first. It's like voluntarily stepping into that desert of effort and uncertainty. But remember the desert leads somewhere. Every day you practice a better habit, every time you challenge an excuse, every time you speak the truth instead of cowering – you are teaching your brain that change is possible, that improvement is happening. And your brain, wonderful machine that it is, will start to heal. New neural pathways will form that reinforce positive behaviors. Your body will respond – maybe your sleep improves, your energy increases, your mood swings level out a bit. Bit by bit, you'll notice you haven't cried in a week where before you cried every day, or you'll realize you genuinely laughed at something, or you'll wake up not dreading the day. These little victories accumulate.

The goal here isn't to eliminate all sadness or anxiety – that's not realistic. It's to build a life that you're mostly happy to be living, and to have the resilience to weather the times when you're not. It's to stop being the biggest obstacle in your own path. The world will throw enough challenges at you; you don't need to be challenging yourself internally on top of that.

In summary, negativity has many faces – the societal kind that breeds intolerance and judgment (like cancel culture), and the personal kind that keeps us stuck in our own dark corners. In both cases, the antidotes are similar: open dialogue, truth, humility, connection, and responsibility. Whether it's engaging with an opposing idea instead of cancelling it, or facing your own issues instead of hiding from them, the path forward lies in confronting the discomfort with courage and honesty.

If you allow it, your mind will surprise you with its capacity to recover, forgive, and find meaning. If you surround yourself with supportive people and also support yourself with good habits, you create an environment where negativity can't easily anchor itself. Life will always have suffering – that's a given. But as Jordan Peterson said, love (for others and oneself) is the desire to reduce unnecessary suffering, and truth is the tool to do it. By speaking up instead of silencing (in society) and by stepping up instead of wallowing (in personal life), we serve the truth, we serve love, and we slowly make things better – both in the world of ideas and within our own skulls. Remember: your brain will heal, if you let it. And "letting it" often means doing the hard things, the unglamorous things, and the scary things – but on the other side of those, there's a life worth living.

Part IV

Healing the Sick Brain

Chapter 9

Purpose, Connection, and Meaning

The Path Is the Purpose

I truly believe that the purpose of life is the path itself. If we were born with everything we needed, then what would we have to chase? Why would we strive, or even bother being social beings? It's the pursuit—each step forward, each first time—that infuses our lives with meaning. I still remember so many of my "firsts" upon arriving in a new country for college. In my freshman year, I would take a two-hour trek on public transportation to the airport at every holiday break, then wait four more hours to board a flight, then spend 15 hours flying home to Brazil (sometimes nearly 24 hours with connections) just to see my family. It was exhausting and exhilarating at the same time, because it was all new. The first time I could afford to call an Uber to the airport instead of navigating buses and trains felt like such a victory to me. It was a simple change, but a huge change. I never took it for granted.

I also remember the first time I went to a rooftop bar in New York City. I felt completely out of place—like I didn't belong there among the glittering lights and chic crowds—but there I was, standing high above the city, part of it. And I remember the first time I splurged on a meal at a restaurant in New York. For two years I had survived on dining hall food (thanks to my scholarship meal plan) and could hardly afford anything else. So that first meal out felt like luxury; I savored every bite and savored the moment of simply being there. If I had been handed all these experiences on a silver platter from the start, would I still feel the same joy and gratitude? Would I have the positive outlook and the grit I carry now? I don't think so. Each of those experiences—no matter how uncomfortable or lengthy or humble—was important. Each step of the journey taught me not to take things for granted.

All of these "firsts" were life-changing in their own ways. Now I look back and marvel at how much has happened in the last four years. So much growth, so many surprises, and it just makes me wonder how much is still yet to come. How much room for growth do I still have?

A lot, I'm sure—and that thought truly excites me. Not because I'm chasing some final result or end point of success (some trophy moment that lasts a day or a week), but because I've learned to enjoy every step that I take. Every small achievement, every new experience—none of it is truly small to me. Maybe the path is what matters most of all.

Breaking Out of the Bubble

I've spoken with people at so many different stages of life, and one thing I know is that perspective is everything. Studying at Columbia gave me a very particular perspective—a "bubble" perspective. Inside the bubble of an elite university, it's easy to lose sight of what life is like for the rest of the world. When I was applying to Columbia, I had big dreams. They weren't tangible or realistic to everyone, but I believed they were reachable for me. Those dreams were always connected to what I could do for society. Even though I don't come from a wealthy family, my goal in life was never simply to "make endless money." Don't get me wrong—money is important, and arguably irreplaceable in many situations. But treating money as the end goal, rather than a means, is a recipe for emptiness in my book. Some people are genuinely happy living comfortably for themselves, and there's no judgment there. But for me, nothing motivates me more than feeling useful, seen, and heard by others. I want to make an impact. We humans are naturally a bit self-centered—each of us is the protagonist of our own story. I'm no different; I want to stand out and be remembered. That desire to be someone fueled my determination from a young age, especially knowing how young I still am and how much time I have ahead to build a meaningful life.

When I got to Columbia, I indeed found many bright-minded individuals. But I also noticed how often we students proclaimed a kind of extreme altruism—talking about how we were going to change the world, fix society, help everyone but ourselves. There was a sense that to be moral or worthy we had to be constantly sacrificing our own needs on the altar of some greater good. Over time, I started to question that mindset. I saw a perverse side to how people preached altruism: it sometimes demanded the sacrifice of one human for another, as if other people's interests should always be placed above your own, denying the value of the individual. According to this view, the "moral" way to live is exclusively for others—an idea that, taken to an extreme, undermines personal freedom, rationality, and independence. I saw the chaos this could lead to: when everyone believes self-sacrifice is the highest good, people start feeling entitled to dictate who should sacrifice and when. High achievers are punished with guilt or forced to yield their hard-earned success to others. It's as if in this bubble, building something for yourself was only okay if you eventually gave it up for someone else.

I slowly embraced a different perspective: one could call it rational self-interest or rational egoism. This means basing your choices on reason, pursuing your own happiness, and valuing your individual life as an end in itself. At first blush, this sounds selfish, I know. But it isn't about being greedy or cruel—it's about recognizing that your life has worth, and you have a right (even a responsibility) to live it fully. In fact, I believe that if more people adopted this mindset, we'd see more genuine kindness in the world, not less. Instead of a culture that glorifies martyrdom and burnout, we'd have one where people help each other voluntarily, out of true generosity, not out of obligation or to appear "good." If I take care of myself and build myself up, I'm in a much better position to lift others up too. In this scenario, acts of kindness and generosity happen freely, with each person's dignity intact—not because someone feels forced to sacrifice their well-being or identity.

Stepping outside the metaphorical bubble also meant staying grounded in reality. I saw classmates get very caught up in campus activism and idealistic projects—sometimes to the point that they lost touch with the actual communities they aimed to serve. Columbia students often talk about grand ideas to fix the world, but I noticed that talk doesn't always translate to understanding the people outside our gates. I never want to fall into that pattern of moralizing from an ivory tower. Real change, I believe, comes from connection and compassion, not from shouting the loudest or flaunting one's virtue. I even saw peers who wrote passionate admissions essays about changing the world end up taking jobs that had nothing to do with those ideals—maybe because reality hit, or maybe because that initial passion wasn't truly theirs. These observations reminded me to always check in with myself: Am I doing this because it's true to my values, or because I'm trying to live up to someone else's idea of "good"?

In short, being in the bubble taught me what I value and what I don't. I value authenticity over appearance. I value using my talents and resources to create value in the world—but in a way that doesn't destroy me in the process. I value kindness, but not the kind that comes from self-neglect or coercion. The institution and its culture challenged me to define my own moral compass. And my compass now points to a philosophy of caring—caring about others and caring about myself. I realized that to truly help anyone, I must never lose myself again.

Freedom in Discipline

One of the greatest lessons I learned during these years is the paradoxical truth that discipline can create freedom. At first glance, freedom and discipline seem at odds—freedom is doing whatever you want, and discipline is doing what you must, right? But I discovered that true freedom isn't about indulging every impulse; it's about having the power to choose what is really good for you, even when your impulses tug the other way.

In my native language (Portuguese), we have a useful distinction between desejo (desire) and vontade (will). Desire is raw, primitive, and often selfish. Will is desire after it's been evaluated by your intellect—it's the filtered desire that aligns with your values and long-term goals. Freedom only truly exists when you are not enslaved by your unfiltered desires. In other words, you become free when you can tell yourself "no" and guide your life with intention. Society today often worships the opposite of discipline in the name of a false freedom—"Do whatever you want, whenever you want; YOLO (you only live once)!" But I learned that constantly giving in to every impulse didn't make me free; it made me a prisoner of whims. There is a real freedom in the ability to pause, evaluate a desire, and sometimes deny it. By passing my urges through the filter of reason—by exercising my vontade—I began to act in ways that served my true well-being, not just my immediate craving.

I had to put this understanding into practice especially during my hardest times. When I was at my lowest, depressed and full of self-doubt, my desejos (desires) were often self-sabotaging: Stay in bed. Skip class. Avoid people. Scroll mindlessly on your phone for hours. Don't eat. Don't move. Those were the easy paths, the primitive impulses born out of pain. My salvation was learning to exert my will instead. I pushed myself to do things that I knew, rationally, would help me, even if I didn't feel like doing them at first. I forced myself to go to sleep at a reasonable hour, because I knew an all-nighter would only deepen my darkness. I dragged myself to the gym when I wanted to hide, because I knew the endorphins would clear some of the fog in my mind. I started cooking and eating nutritious food again, even when I had no appetite, because I understood my brain chemistry needed those building blocks. Each time I acted out of will rather than passing desire, I was reclaiming a bit of freedom from the monster of depression. It was not easy—honestly, it was like fighting a part of myself—but it was liberating in the end. I was no longer obeying every negative voice in my head. I was choosing what to obey and what to ignore.

I even adopted a counterintuitive little strategy during this period: do well what you hate to do. If I had a task I truly loathed, I challenged myself to tackle it with excellence. For example, if I dreaded a particular class assignment or a bureaucratic chore, I would pour extra effort into it. It sounds strange, but by doing that, I often found I only had to do it once (because I got it right) or I discovered aspects of it that weren't so bad after all. In a way, this was another exercise of willpower—refusing to do a half-hearted job even on things I didn't like. It gave me a sense of control: rather than the task mastering me (through procrastination or poor performance), I mastered the task. And once it was done well, I could move on without that burden hanging over me. This mindset turned many unpleasant duties into opportunities for pride and learning.

Hand in hand with discipline came the lesson of self-care. Earlier in college, I had fallen into the trap of trying to do everything and be everything for everyone. I thought saying "yes" to every project, every opportunity, every person in need was the right thing to do—after all, isn't that what a driven, altruistic student is supposed to do? But spreading myself so thin only made me ineffective and miserable. I burned out hard. I developed an unhealthy relationship with food, with sleep, with my own body. There came a point where I simply couldn't focus or muster motivation; I was done. It was a rude awakening, but an important one: I realized that I am not limitless. No one is. We all have limits, and respecting them is not weakness—it's wisdom.

A fellow student once shared a brilliant analogy with me that illustrates this well: Advocacy is like brushing your teeth. Imagine each issue you care about is a tooth in your mouth. Some are front and center, some are hidden in the back, but you need to "brush" all of them to keep the whole mouth healthy. Now, when we're passionate, we try to tackle every issue—we brush every tooth diligently. But what happens if you brush and brush and never pause? Your toothbrush wears out. You wear out. The toothbrush in this analogy is you—your mind, your body, your spirit. If you don't take care of the toothbrush, pretty soon you won't be able to brush anything at all. This image struck me deeply. I realized I had worn my own "bristles" down to nothing. I had to step back and take care of the tool—take care of myself—if I wanted to do any good for others in the long run.

From then on, I started viewing self-care as an integral part of my mission, not as an optional indulgence. I began to practice saying "no" when I knew I didn't have the bandwidth. I allowed myself to sleep more, to take breaks, to eat meals on time, to simply breathe. I let go of the toxic expectation that I had to be perfect or accomplish everything by myself. I even went to therapy and learned how to be kinder to the person in the mirror. And you know what? By healing myself, by recharging my own battery, I actually became more effective in everything I did choose to do. I showed up for my friends in a genuine way. I improved in my coursework. I had the energy to start new initiatives that truly mattered to me. It was as if by saving myself, I regained the power to help save others.

This was a revelation: we cannot help anyone if we are running on empty. We cannot "fight the good fight" in the world if we've declared war on our own bodies or minds. True altruism includes caring for the self. I had to learn that the hard way, but I'm grateful I did. Going forward, this balance—discipline, self-care, and mindful choices—is something I carry like precious armor. It's what will allow me to keep walking my path without losing myself again.

Stories That Shaped My Calling

In the fall of my junior year, life tested me with one of the hardest experiences I've ever faced. It began with a knock on my dorm room door one night. I opened it to find my close friend, Giovanna, standing there. It was early September, classes had just begun, and I was at my desk buried in readings, full of the usual excitement and jitters of a new semester. But the look on Giovanna's face stopped me cold. She came in and leaned against the wall, uncharacteristically quiet.

"Sometimes I think about it," she said softly, almost in a whisper. "About what, amiga?" I turned to her, sensing something was wrong. Giovanna raised her hand and pointed two fingers to her temple, mimicking a gun. Then she made a small "poof" sound with her mouth. In that instant, I felt my stomach drop. The smile that had been on my face vanished, and my heart began to pound so loudly I could hear it in my ears. My smartwatch even vibrated on my wrist, alerting me of an elevated heart rate—my body knew before my mind fully did that this was serious. She was telling me she sometimes thought about killing herself.

I took a few seconds, just breathing, trying to remain calm though inside I was anything but. I gently guided Giovanna to sit down next to me on my narrow dorm bed, and I wrapped my arms around her in a tight hug. "Gi, listen to me," I said, my voice shaking despite my efforts to steady it. "What you just told me is very serious. I can't let you carry that alone—and I can't carry it alone either. I won't. We're going to get help, okay? We're going to a psychiatrist together, you and me."

Giovanna stiffened and pulled back. "What? Just because I suggested I think about...that? Come on. A psych isn't going to help," she argued, trying to downplay it. I could hear the defensiveness, the fear under her flippant tone. We went back and forth for a while. I pleaded, I reasoned, I even threatened (lightly) that I'd have to involve someone if she wouldn't see a professional. Finally, she agreed to go talk to someone—but only if I let her do it alone. She didn't want me or anyone else "babysitting" her through it.

Reluctantly, I respected her wish. I checked in with her constantly over the next days and weeks. She said she was "fine." She had, in fact, seen a campus counselor once. She insisted that she didn't want to make a big deal of it. I tried to be hopeful, but a knot of worry lived in my stomach those weeks. I told a resident advisor generally that a friend was in a bad place (without naming her, since she'd asked for privacy), and I got some advice—but there's only so much others can do if the person herself doesn't want help.

Four weeks after that night in my dorm, Giovanna took her own life. When I got the news, I felt like the world stopped. I couldn't breathe. I couldn't process how the sun was still rising and setting, how people were still going to class and complaining about midterms, while my dear friend had been in such darkness and was now…gone. I replayed our conversation a thousand times in my head, tormenting myself with What if's. What if I had dragged her to the hospital that night? What if I had sat in on her counselling session? What if I had alerted her parents, her siblings, someone? A wave of guilt and grief unlike anything I'd known before crashed over me.

I thought I understood something about death and loss before this. When I was 11, my godmother—a woman I loved dearly—died by suicide (an overdose of medication). I remember standing at her funeral, stunned and confused, and then turning to comfort my own mother in her grief. Even as a child, I stepped into the role of supporter, trying to be strong for others. Perhaps I thought that experience had taught me how to handle loss. But losing Giovanna proved that I still had so much to learn. I still didn't really know how to deal with death—especially a death like this, sudden, preventable, and clouded by the painful haze of mental illness.

At the same time I lost Giovanna, I was fighting battles of my own. I was an immigrant far from home, trying to navigate life in a different language and culture. I was pushing myself through a full course load at one of the most demanding schools in the country. And I was trying to pretend I had it all together, even as depression was constantly lurking at my door. There were days I felt like I was barely keeping my head above water—and then here came a tidal wave to pull me under. It would have been so easy to give up entirely at that point, to become bitter or hopeless. A part of me was very tempted to.

And yet, amid that despair, something became clearer than ever: why I needed to continue on the path to becoming a doctor. After Giovanna's death, some people gently asked me if I was sure I wanted to go into such a tough, emotionally taxing field as medicine. They knew I had been through a lot. They worried I might be choosing it for the wrong reasons, or that it might break me further. I asked myself the same thing: Why, after all of this pain, do I still want to go to medical school?

The answer that rose from deep inside me was simple: Because I am passionate about stories. By "stories," I mean the lives and experiences of people: people like Giovanna, people like my godmother, people like me. I want to be a doctor because every patient is a story, and those stories need and deserve better endings. I realized that what truly draws me to medicine isn't the prestige or the white coat or even the intellectual challenge (though I do love the science); it's the human connection. It's being able to step into someone's life at their most vulnerable moment and help them rewrite a frightening chapter into one of hope or healing. Medicine, to me, is storytelling in its highest form: it's taking the narrative of illness or injury and guiding it toward healing and meaning.

I have countless little examples that reaffirm this passion. I remember the rush of right certainty I felt when I diagnosed my young cousin Ana's appendicitis at a family gathering—recognizing the symptoms early, urging that we get her to a hospital, and later hearing the doctors say, "Good thing she came in when she did." I remember helping a close friend through an eating disorder, spending nights by her side, researching treatment options, encouraging her bite by bite—celebrating every tiny victory in her recovery. I remember bringing another friend with crippling anxiety to the gym with me, and over weeks seeing that exercise and routine brought some light back into his eyes. I can't forget running a half-marathon and being acutely aware, with every stride, of how my body was converting stored calories into energy (thank you, biochemistry!) and how the burning in my legs was lactic acid buildup—not a signal to stop, but a sign that I was getting stronger. That knowledge comforted me and pushed me onward. I think of moments with my family: patiently explaining to my grandmother that her arthritis does not steal away her identity—she is still the same vibrant person, just dealing with a stubborn joint disease. Or the many times I have carefully gone over the dangers of smoking with my mother, hoping one day she'll decide to quit for good. Or the afternoons spent playing crossword puzzles with my grandpa to help keep his mind sharp, because I know the value of these cognitive exercises in staving off dementia. These might sound like small things—just helping friends and family—but to me, this is medicine in action. It's woven into my life. Every time I share knowledge, every time I alleviate someone's worry or encourage a healthier choice, I feel that spark. I feel this is what I'm meant to do.

More than anything, I want to be a physician because, in a very real sense, medicine saved me. When I was drowning in depression, I clung to the idea that I could still be useful to someone tomorrow. On days I planned to give up, I would tell myself, "Not today. Because maybe tomorrow a friend will need me, and I have to be there for them." That thought kept me alive. And each time I did help someone, it pulled me back from the ledge a little more. The purpose I found in caring for others became the lifeline that guided me out of my own darkness. In those moments, it didn't matter that I wasn't a licensed doctor—I was already practicing the core of medicine: compassion, presence, knowledge-sharing, healing.

I remember feeling already a doctor the day I convinced my own father not to drink and drive. I had noticed the pattern of his behavior, and I sat him down and pleaded from the bottom of my heart, armed with statistics and heartfelt words, that he must stop this before a tragedy happened. The relief and pride I felt when he actually changed his habits was immense. It was the first time I felt the weight of potentially saving a life—a life very dear to me—through persistent caring and truthful counsel. It struck me: This is what a doctor can do. It's not always about scalpels and prescriptions; often it's about tough conversations and earning trust and guiding someone toward a safer path.

Not long after, I had another formative experience that solidified my calling. I spent a summer volunteering in a rural community in Piauí, one of the poorest regions in Brazil. There, I saw first-hand what lack of access to healthcare does to people. I met children who were years behind on vaccines, mothers who walked miles under the sun to get basic medicines, and elders who endured chronic pain with stoic grace because there were no doctors around consistently to help them. It broke my heart, but it also lit a fire in me. Serving that underserved community showed me that the skills and knowledge I aim to gain as a doctor could directly, tangibly improve lives that were hanging in the balance. In Piauí, I confirmed my decision to become not just any doctor, but one who works in the places and with the people who need it most. The role of a physician, as I witnessed there, goes far beyond treating symptoms—it's about being an advocate, a problem-solver, sometimes a one-person safety net for an entire village. It's about caring in the broadest sense: caring for individuals, caring for communities, caring enough to fight inequity and injustice in health. I realized the doctor I aspire to be is equal parts caregiver, advocate, and scientist. That role aligns perfectly with my core values of compassion, service, and curiosity.

Every story—my own, Giovanna's, my family's, those patients in Piauí—has shaped my path to service. They've taught me that illness is not just a malfunction of body parts; it's a story of a person, often a story of suffering, that cries out to be heard and understood. They've taught me that sometimes all it takes is one person who truly listens and cares to change the entire trajectory of someone's life. I know I can't save everyone. I couldn't save Giovanna, and I will always carry that sorrow with me. But I also carry with me the determination that in the future, I will be that person who stays present, who asks the hard questions, who offers help again and again, even if it's initially refused. I want to be the doctor who sees a patient as a whole person—mind, body, and soul. I want to be the one who can say, "I know it hurts. I'm here with you. Let's find a way through this, together."

I am passionate about stories, especially the ones that are mired in pain, because I have lived through pain and I have seen how the story can change. I want to devote my life to changing those stories, to making life worth living in the face of death and despair. That is my purpose, as clear as day now, forged by everything I've lived through.

Was Columbia Worth It?

A question I've turned over in my head many times: Was Columbia worth it? Was it worth the pain, the stress, the sleepless nights, the homesickness, the self-doubt? After all that I've recounted—the depression, the struggles—did this prestigious education justify its price, both literal and figurative? My answer, honestly, is yes. Yes, it was worth it, but not for the obvious reasons. It wasn't worth it because of the fancy classes or the Nobel laureate professors or the gleaming resume bullet points. Those things are nice, but they're not what made it worthwhile. Columbia was worth it because of the person it forced me to become.

In the past four years, I learned more about the world and myself than I ever imagined I would. Sure, I gained knowledge—I learned about Plato and proteins, Baudelaire and black holes, calculus and community health. But more importantly, I gained perspective. I met people from every corner of the globe, with beliefs and backgrounds vastly different from mine. I learned to appreciate cultures and viewpoints I'd never encountered back home. I stepped outside my comfort zone again and again. Each time, I discovered a new piece of myself.

What did I learn at Columbia University? I learned that to truly take care of others, I must also take care of myself. I learned that intellect alone isn't everything; character and kindness count for far more. I learned that success is hollow if it comes at the cost of your well-being or integrity. And I learned, above all, that I am resilient and capable of change. I came to Columbia somewhat broken (though I didn't realize it then), and I left more whole. I left healed in many ways. I had left my country at 17 in search of an education and perhaps in search of myself. I found both. I found me. The price of that self-discovery included many tears and hard nights, but it's a price I would pay again because the reward is my life. I am alive, and I want to live. For a while, I couldn't say that with confidence. Now I can. So yes, it was worth it. And if you're wondering—yes, you can heal too. If I could do it, anyone can; I truly believe that.

Ironically, one of the turning points in my Columbia journey was when I started caring less about Columbia. Let me explain: In my freshman and part of sophomore year, I was consumed by the academic pressure. I tied my entire self-worth to grades and performance. Columbia was this towering institution and I was constantly terrified of not measuring up. My depression fed on that fear. It told me I was an imposter, that Columbia had made a mistake in admitting me. I remember nights lying awake in my dorm room, staring at the ceiling, thinking of ways to apologize for my very existence. Should I email the admissions office and tell them they were wrong? Should I drop out quietly before I mess up their statistics? Should I… just disappear so I don't disappoint anyone anymore? These thoughts were dark, and they were relentless. Depression is a cruel liar, and it had convinced me that I was worthless, that nothing I did mattered, that I'd never catch up to the brilliance around me.

I was so afraid of failing that I nearly failed to live. My worst moment was when I felt death might be a relief—a way to stop pretending, a way to stop being a burden. That's how distorted my thinking had become. On the outside, maybe I just seemed like a tired, apathetic student who didn't care as much as others about an upcoming exam or paper. People might have seen me skipping study sessions or not freaking out like everyone else and thought, "Wow, she's so laid-back. She doesn't care." But inside, I cared too much—I cared to the point that it paralyzed me. It wasn't that I had some zen confidence; I had despair. It made me appear calm in a twisted way, because I had already imagined the worst outcome and resigned myself to it. Depression can look like indifference, but it's actually defeat.

The change began in the latter half of sophomore year. There was a tiny spark inside me—a voice that wasn't entirely drowned out—that whispered: This is not how your story is going to end. Call it survival instinct, call it divine grace, call it sheer stubbornness—something made me get up one day and say, "Enough." I was still alive, and as long as I was alive, I owed it to myself to try. If I was going to quit anything, I was going to quit being so cruel to myself. If I was going to give up something, I would give up trying to be perfect for once. I decided, almost experimentally, to prioritize feeling okay over doing everything.

I started to let myself sleep at a normal time. At first, it was because I literally couldn't stay awake—my body was at its limit. But then I made it a rule: no more all-nighters unless absolutely necessary (and honestly, in most cases, they aren't truly necessary). I reconnected with exercise, gingerly at first. I remember telling myself, "Well, if I can't be the top student, maybe I can at least have a healthy body. Maybe I can be strong physically, since I feel so weak mentally." So I went to the gym regularly. I lifted weights, I ran on the treadmill, I did those things consistently, almost religiously, because it was one thing in my life that had a clear, positive outcome. If you lift weights, you will get stronger—maybe not immediately, but eventually. That simple cause-and-effect was comforting when nothing else in life felt under my control.

I also began to pay attention to what I was feeding myself—both my body and my mind. I had fallen into poor eating habits (some days I'd eat nothing but junk; other days I'd practically starve then binge), and that wreaked havoc not just on my body but on my mood. As I studied some neuroscience and psychology in class, I started applying it to myself. I learned about neurotransmitters like serotonin and dopamine, the chemicals that regulate mood. I realized that I had been depleting them or throwing them out of balance with my erratic habits. For instance, the quick dopamine hits from endless social media scrolling were only making me more miserable after the brief distraction wore off. So I cut back dramatically on my screen time, especially on apps that weren't actually bringing me real joy or knowledge. Instead, I sought dopamine in more natural ways: exercise (there it is again), spending time outdoors, listening to music I loved. I sought serotonin by eating better and yes, by forcing myself to interact with friends even when I felt low, because positive social interactions boost serotonin. Bit by bit, these small changes started adding up. I could feel a shift—like I had been at the bottom of a deep, dark pool, and I was slowly floating upward toward the light. One of the most powerful things I did was reconnect with my childhood passions. I asked myself, When was the last time I remember being truly happy, light-hearted, myself? My mind flew back to my childhood, before all the pressure hit. As a child I loved dancing, painting, singing, writing silly stories—none of it for achievement, all of it for pure pleasure. Children have a way of living in the moment and doing what feels good for the soul. So I decided to let my inner child take the reins sometimes. I started dancing again—sometimes just in my dorm room, earbuds in, dancing like a fool and laughing, sometimes by taking a Zumba or hip-hop class at the student center. I dug out an old sketchbook and began to draw and paint, with absolutely zero intention of showing anyone my art or being "good" at it. I attended open-mic nights and poetry readings, something I'd stopped doing after freshman year stole my free time. I even joined a student choir for a semester, because I remembered how much joy singing used to bring me. These things were magical. They didn't solve my problems overnight, but they gave me moments—moments of peace, moments of genuine happiness, moments where I thought, Hey, there you are. There's the girl I remember. Each of those moments was like collecting shiny little stones that I could hold in my pocket to remind myself life could still sparkle.

Simultaneously, I addressed the more serious aspect of my health: I acknowledged that I had developed an eating disorder amidst all the chaos. Controlling my food had become a way to cope when everything else felt out of control. With the help of a campus counselor and a lot of honest introspection, I worked on healing that relationship with food. Weightlifting, interestingly, played a positive role here too. It taught me to see food as fuel for my muscles and brain. I started respecting my body's needs instead of punishing it. The more I learned about the science of nutrition and exercise, the more I was able to silence the irrational voice that wanted to deprive or harm my body. I replaced "I need to be skinny" with "I want to be strong"—strong enough to lift heavy weights, strong enough to carry myself through long days, strong enough to save lives one day. That mindset shift was liberating and healing.

By the time junior year rolled around, I moved into a single room. Living alone was a test of everything I had implemented. There was no roommate to pull me out of bed if I overslept, no built-in daily human interaction to fall back on. It was just me and me. I won't lie—at first I was a little worried. Would loneliness creep in and undo my progress? But I framed it differently: this was my chance to prove that I could take full responsibility for myself. I treated myself almost like my own child or my own patient. I established routines to keep me healthy: I stuck to my regular sleep schedule; I meal-prepped on Sundays; I penciled in gym sessions as if they were important classes (because they were important appointments with my well-being). I also kept an eye on my thoughts, journaling often to catch any negative spirals before they got out of hand. Living alone turned out to be one of the best experiences for my growth. I found that I actually enjoyed my own company. I could spend a Friday night painting or watching a movie without feeling "lame" or guilty for not socializing or studying nonstop. I had finally achieved a balance that worked for me—academics, social life, self-care, all in harmony (well, more harmony than before, at least).

So, was Columbia worth it? Yes, a thousand times yes, but not for Columbia's sake—for mine. Columbia was the crucible in which I shattered, yes, but also the one in which I was re-forged stronger. I entered that school thinking Columbia was some almighty entity I had to appease. I left realizing Columbia is just a place, an institution made up of humans, like any other. I am the one who has to live with myself forever, not with Columbia. In fact, I came to see that I am larger than the institution in the sense that my life and my identity can't be confined to it. Columbia is one chapter of my story, not the whole book. The university exists to serve students and society, not for students to serve it or worship it. This perspective was freeing.

I look around at the debate nowadays: some people advocate skipping college altogether, others insist that without a degree you have no future in this competitive world. To me, both viewpoints miss the point. The real question is, what do you want out of life and how will you get it? College can be an amazing tool or a destructive force—it depends on how you use it and what you expect from it. My goal in life isn't a title or a salary; my goal is to live a life of meaning, to serve others and enjoy the journey along the way. Education can absolutely further that goal—learning skills, gaining knowledge, meeting inspiring people can all amplify your ability to contribute to the world. But if you go into college without a strong sense of self, it can also derail you. You might get swept up by the rat race of GPA, internships, prestige, and forget why you started in the first place. I was fortunate (or unfortunate) to face a crisis of self early on; it forced me to define what truly mattered to me. Not everyone has that moment of clarity, and it's easy to lose yourself in the chase for accolades. I see it happen often: a classmate would get an amazing internship but be miserable because it wasn't actually what they wanted; another would win some academic prize but at the cost of their mental health. Society might label those outcomes "success," but I've learned to question that. Success, to me, is being healthy, happy, and helpful to others.

Only a very few people in this world will become a Mozart or a Marie Curie or an Elon Musk—those once-in-a-generation figures who redefine fields. Chasing that kind of singular greatness can drive you mad because it's not something you can plan or guarantee with hard work alone. I've made peace with that. I don't need to be a Mozart; I just need to be myself and make the best out of the talents and opportunities I have. If I can leave a positive mark on the people I meet and the community I serve, that is a legacy enough. In fact, the world doesn't need every one of us to be a prodigy; the world needs people who are kind, ethical, and passionate in the everyday as well. That's something I think Columbia (and places like it) should teach more of: how to be a good person, not just a good test-taker.

As I prepare to graduate and move on to medical school, I carry these hard-won lessons close to my heart. I sometimes joke with my friends with phrases like, "You can only dream big if you sleep well," or "So, you want to save lives? Have you tried saving yours first?" They laugh, and I laugh, but I'm also being quite serious. These are truths I'll never again ignore. I will make sure to get my sleep, because I know my dreams (literally and figuratively) depend on it. I will take care of my own health, because I've seen what happens when I don't, and because I owe that to any future patients—how dare I try to fix someone else's life if my own is in shambles? It's like the airplane safety briefing: put on your own oxygen mask before assisting others. I've finally learned the wisdom in that.

Now, on the brink of a new chapter, I don't have all the answers about who exactly I will become. I have some goals, sure. I see a vision of Dr. Nicole, serving in underprivileged communities, perhaps blending clinical practice with public health advocacy, maybe even bringing arts and music into healing. But life is full of twists, and I'm okay with that. I do know, however, who I do not want to become. I refuse to become someone who stops listening to others, or someone who loses empathy. I refuse to become a person who neglects her family or friends or forgets where she came from. I refuse to be a hypocrite who tells people to live healthy while secretly self-destructing. I refuse to be "useless" to society in the sense of living only for myself without contributing goodness to the world around me. As long as I keep not being those things, I think I'll turn out alright in whatever I do.

Sometimes I think about life as a grand improvisation. You can plan and plan, make battle plans for every step (and believe me, I tried), but inevitably something will go wrong. Often, many things will go wrong. And that's okay. I've learned to adapt, to be flexible and even find humor in the failures. There is a popular saying: "When life gives you lemons, make lemonade." One of my friends improved on it: "When life gives you lemons, slice them up, grab some salt, and take a tequila shot!" In short, if you stop seeing life's surprises and setbacks as your enemies, you can often turn them into adventures. I'm no longer scared of detours and lemons. Some of the best things in my life came from detours I never intended to take.

How do I go on from here? I go on with faith in the path. I don't see the end of college as the peak of my life or as the end of anything really; it's just the end of a chapter. My story continues, and its purpose continues to be something I forge day by day. I've come to understand that meaning isn't something waiting for us at the finish line, like a trophy. Meaning is something we create in each moment, with each choice and each connection. My life's purpose is not a fixed destination or a specific achievement; my purpose is to walk this journey as fully and as authentically as I can.

I know there will be challenges ahead, as life will inevitably bring new hardships. I also know there will be incredible joys: new friendships, the first time I save a life or deliver a baby or comfort someone in despair, the day I wear that white coat for real. I will embrace it all. The ups and the downs. The meaning of life, to me, is found in that rich tapestry of experiences. It's in the way we respond, the lessons we learn, the love we give and receive along the way.

So, as I step forward, I carry a piece of wisdom that I earned through these years: The purpose of life is the path. Stay present. Stay hopeful. Take care of yourself so you can care for others. Cherish the people around you. Be grateful for the smallest things. Keep walking, keep learning. Sometimes you'll stumble, sometimes you'll dance, sometimes you'll crawl. Just don't quit. If you're in a dark place, hold on: the light will return, I promise. If you're in a good place, savour it: these moments are the precious fuel that will keep you going when times get tough again.

This is how I choose to go on from here: with my past acknowledged, my present embraced, and my future open. With humility, with curiosity, with courage, and with the understanding that every day, every step, is in itself the meaning of life. That is what makes life worth living, and that is what I'm carrying with me as I continue down this beautiful, unpredictable path.

www.ingramcontent.com/pod-product-compliance
Lightning Source LLC
Chambersburg PA
CBHW042335050426
PP18089900001B/1